ADVENTURES OF A
ONE-BREASTED WOMAN

BOOKSMYTH PRESS

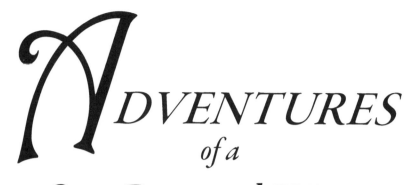

Adventures
of a
One-Breasted Woman

RECLAIMING MY MOXIE
AFTER CANCER

SUSAN CUMMINGS

Booksmyth Press
Shelburne Falls, Massachusetts

Printed in the United States of America

ISBN: 978-0-9815830-7-5

Library of Congress Control Number 2012914780

Book design by Maureen Moore

Illustrations and photograph by Susan Cummings

This is a memoir. However, a few people have been
disguised to protect their privacy. Also, maybe my
memory could have been better sometimes.

Published by Booksmyth Press
Shelburne Falls, MA 01370
www.thebooksmyth.com

IN MEMORY OF

Diana, Karen and J

What blazes the trail is not necessarily pretty.

Mary Oliver, "Skunk Cabbage"

CONTENTS ❦

ADVENTURES OF A
ONE-BREASTED WOMAN

1 ✑

Adventures, Some Chosen

I HAD A CHOICE AFTER I GRADUATED FROM THE UNI-versity of Colorado. I had planned to continue in school to earn my credentials to teach high school English, but then I was offered a Ford Foundation Fellowship to teach English as a Second Language at the American University in Cairo. Choosing took a nanosecond.

Egypt provided almost nonstop adventures. My day job gave me many a peak moment, such as trying to explain to my wide-eyed students, with ever more gesticulation, the versa-tility of the words "lie," "lay" and "lying." After-work hours proved even more interesting. It was 1968, shortly after the Arab-Israeli Six-Day War. Virtually no tourists were venturing into Egypt, and President Gamal Abdel Nasser didn't permit foreign journalists. I saw this as an opportunity to write sev-eral freelance newspaper articles about postwar Cairo, which I convinced a brave traveler to smuggle out of the country. For this attempt at being an intrepid foreign correspondent, I could have been deported. Both the brave traveler and I could have been thrown into one of Nasser's notorious jails. Other enlivening extracurricular activities included encouraging the interest of a dashing young Egyptian computer programmer while deflecting his intention to sleep with me; straining my middle-class, suburban New York mind to fathom why and how the mammoth necropolises at Giza and the Valley of the Kings were built; and scuba diving amidst the teeming psychedelic life of the Red Sea. One day I got the sun-baked idea to hitchhike *alone* from Alexandria to Mersa Matruh, a resort town further east along the Mediterranean coast. Luckily the two English-speaking government workers who picked me up were more interested in friendly chat than, say, rape.

My high-risk undertakings did manage to evoke a slight amount of fear in my addled young mind, but the fear only egged me on, sharpened my senses. Fear is an integral part of many adventures: a little adds to the thrill. Too much fear, though, and you become paralyzed.

Twenty-four years later, for example, in 1992, I was sure the technician was going to peek into the tiny dressing cubicle where I sat in a flimsy hospital gown and say, as usual, "Everything's fine, Miss Cummings. You can get dressed and go home." I was giddy. It was a late winter afternoon in New York City, gray but unseasonably warm, with the slightest promise of daffodils in the air. Even more exciting, just as I was leaving my apartment on East Eighty-second Street to go downtown for my yearly mammogram appointment in Greenwich Village, the phone rang. It was the actress who had played sweet Annelle, with me as cantankerous Ouiser, in a three-week run of *Steel Magnolias* in Brooklyn. I thought Sylvia was calling to kid me because on one of my entrances in our last show, the day before, I had massacred my line. Apparently I had maneuvered past this blooper successfully because she said her agent had been in the audience and had asked if I would call him!

The technician at the breast cancer screening center peeked in. "After you dress, the doctor wants to see you in his office."

My mammograms must reveal something fascinating, benignly so of course, I thought, and the doctor wants to share this with me. I didn't have the slightest worry about breast cancer. No one I knew of in my family had had the disease, and I was the smallest-breasted woman I knew. Where would cancer have room to grow? I had regarded going for my mammograms for the past seven years as an administrative chore—momentarily excruciating, to be sure, wherein my little peas were squeezed into lilliputian pancakes, but also validating. Despite my minimalist frontal features, I was still womanly, still in the club of the rest of my female friends over forty who had their breasts monitored.

A gorgeous, brown-skinned man with straight, shiny, black hair swished into the sterile white room. He was about my age, I noted, definitely taller than my five feet nine and a half inches, slim like me, and the critical finger on his left hand was unencumbered.

"Miss Cummings, you have highly suspicious micro-calcifications in your left breast."

With his singsongy, delicately clipped Indian accent, this bomb to my brain seemed to be exploding during a raga concert. My left leg started shaking up and down like a jackhammer. Sweat streamed from my armpits. "Isn't calcium a good thing?" I squeaked.

"Micro-calcifications are highly suspicious of breast cancer."

"In a breast that isn't even double-A?"

"Breast size has nothing to do with it, Miss Cummings. I could be wrong—I hope I am—but I suggest you get a biopsy as soon as possible."

I had no more questions for the doctor. I could no longer

speak. A black cloud filled my body. I floated into the waiting room, where the cloud let loose a storm of tears.

I didn't call the agent.

I did what I was told. I had no choice.

"I'm so sorry, Miss Cummings, the biopsy is not negative," is the way my surgeon at Memorial Sloan-Kettering Cancer Center put it—thus avoiding referring to cancer as "positive"—when she phoned in early March 1992. The biopsy revealed cancer in my milk ducts, ductal carcinoma in situ (DCIS), Dr. S said.

I was standing holding the phone by my kitchen table, dressed in my white terrycloth robe, jeans and sneakers. Still recuperating from the biopsy, I was about ready to venture out to Central Park. Its quiet browns and greens and reflective waters buffered the bustling Upper East Side of the city from the bustling Upper West Side, always giving me solace. My stomach clenched like teeth at her news, while the rest of my body felt empty, limp.

I didn't make it to the park. After my surgeon and I said good-bye, I laid my right hand lightly over the left side of my robe. The tape that held the bandage in place was pulling my skin, but I didn't adjust it. I didn't dare disturb a cell. I staggered the two feet to my filing cabinet and leaned against it. It was white. The kitchen walls were white. I was engulfed in white, hospital white.

Cancer, I definitely had cancer. *I* had *cancer.* I might die at forty-seven.

I knew what would happen if I did. My older sister, breathtakingly efficient, would take a taxi across Central Park from her family's apartment on West 107th Street and manage the emptying of my apartment. Nancy would whip through my five drawers of files in less than thirty minutes, throwing all the files into black plastic garbage bags, except perhaps the ones labeled "Money Matters" and "Insurance." That's how it would be. I knew because we had cleaned out our mother's apartment together four years earlier after she had died of lung cancer. I didn't blame my sister. What did I expect her to do with the remnants of my unfinished life?

I took a step back, pulled out the top drawer of the cabinet, glanced at the file labels and slammed it shut. I opened the next drawer—slam. The files contained mementos only I considered precious: my diploma from Dorothy's Play School in 1949, with the red and white candy cane border; my scuba diving certificate, for which I took a course three years *after* my dives in the Red Sea; letters and cards from friends and family. I'd saved unremarkable things, really: records of the attempts of our tenants' group to rid our block of drug dealers on East Tenth Street, where I'd lived for ten years before moving to staid but safer East Eighty-second; transcripts of more or less helpful sessions with tea leaf, tarot card and planet readers, none of whom told me I'd get cancer. Did any of them know?

I pulled out another drawer, slammed it and slumped back against the cabinet. The files were a record of my life *so far*: newspaper articles I'd written for *The Northern Virginia Sun* after I'd returned from the Middle East, my MS in environmental engineering from Berkeley, environmental reports from my stints at various consulting firms, my songs for various cabaret acts, favorite acting monologues. I hadn't yet tried my folder of ideas for meeting that illusive special someone. I doubled over, dry heaving.

On the one hand, Dr. S consoled me at my next appointment, I was very lucky since DCIS was the earliest form of breast cancer, stage zero. It was still confined to my milk ducts. On the other hand, she and other doctors whom I consulted warned, my cancer cells were the "comedo" type, which grew very aggressively. I had a choice of treatments: a lumpectomy followed by radiation or a mastectomy. While the latter alternative would be more disfiguring, it would also be a somewhat more assured cure, they said.

Within a month, on April 3, 1992, I had a mastectomy.

That was the end of my treatment. My surgeon told me I had about a 99 percent chance of never having a recurrence. Hearing this, many women would have said a million thankyous to their archetype of good fortune and moved on with the rest of their lives.

"YOU'RE OVER-ACTING!" THE DRAMA TEACHER YELLED when I was in my twenties. Humiliated, devastated, I never returned to her workshop and didn't take up acting again for over a decade.

I've been known to overact, overreact, overdo.

I DIDN'T MOVE ON AFTER MY mastectomy. I suppose I had a choice here, but I didn't recognize it. For several years, I couldn't even audition, which, as a New York actress, I'd previously been spending most of my time doing. I was like a deer trapped in a circle of glaring headlights. I could have died. I still might. I could be among that 1 percent who get a recurrence. I was even more frightened when several doctors informed me that cancer survivors are at increased risk for getting other cancers and that this risk increases every year. I was also terrified of living. What kind of life, especially love life, could I expect as a single woman progressing at lightning speed through her middle years, who was now one-breasted and carried the stigma of having had cancer? I obsessed about the cause and the fact of the altered shape of my body for over six years.

What, you may ask, could I possibly have been doing all this time? When I was diagnosed, I had a part-time clerkship at a gastroenterologist's—about as glamorous as a colonoscopy—

to pay for niceties like the rent while I pursued acting. But after my diagnosis, much, sometimes all, of the rest of my spare time was spent not acting, but having adventures of a very different kind. I didn't recognize them as adventures at the time, but the word adventure is derived from the Latin *advenire*, to arrive, and each of my adventures did take me to a new place.

Most of these adventures began by my wanting something. Despite my height and my bushy dark brown hair, I think I often resembled a basset hound in my dogged pursuit, nose to the ground, floppy ears blocking out all save the craved scent. I sought so much—outlets for my fear of and anger at cancer, more beauty in life, some beauty in me. I needed a health plan that would absolutely guarantee I would never, ever get cancer again. I wanted to somehow give back for all the kindness and love I received after diagnosis and during and after treatment. I needed a new kind of faith. I wanted to dance. And maybe possibly somehow someday even find someone to dance with? I wanted my moxie back.

I wouldn't have chosen breast cancer in a million years. I wouldn't have chosen the adventures that followed either, but now, as absurdly romantic as this may seem, I look back at most of them with gratitude, fondness even. They were sometimes scary, sometimes very painful, but often fascinating, lovely, a hoot. Some broke my heart, but they must have broken it more open because my heart seems bigger now. I would pursue each of my adventures until I found satisfaction—the basset must have her bone. And along the way, I discovered possibilities in me and for my life that had previously seemed out of the question.

Every breast cancer survivor walks her own path. My heart will never stop aching for the countless women, several dear friends, who fought the disease in every way they could and lost. *When* will there be a cure for this scourge! In my case, cancer was discovered very early, treatment was severe and wrenching but relatively simple and quick, and so far I am well. Also, as I say, my responses to things can tend toward over-the-top. Still, I hope this book will lighten the way for others— provide a little trail mix, a slightly twisted walking stick.

2 ॐ

Because

I GOT BREAST CANCER BECAUSE MY MENSTRUAL CYCLE started early, at age eleven.

No, I got it because I was a tomboy until eleven so I confused my hormones.

No, I got it because at eleven I let my girlfriends convince me to stop being a tomboy.

No, I got it because at sixteen I had a dermoid cyst on one of my ovaries, and when the surgeon was removing it, he decided to go ahead and cut out the entire ovary as well.

Did I get it because I took birth control pills for five years in my twenties?

I got it because, though I did get pregnant once, I never had a baby.

No relative I know of had breast cancer.

I got it because I worked for a consulting firm on the ninetieth floor of 2 World Trade Center, under fluorescent lights, by windows you couldn't open, for ten years. I did have a great boss though, who encouraged my early forays into cabaret and theatre.

I got it because my body became a hazardous waste dump from all the pollutants I must have breathed in through the years—smog, acid rain, particulates, fumes from the dry cleaner, the volatile solvents in housecleaning products. Well, I hardly ever cleaned. What about the skin products with ingredient lists that would stump a chemist? And the food additives "generally recognized as safe" by the FDA? Why didn't the FDA regulate to increase *my* shelf-life?

Maybe I got cancer because of the fumes I breathed while painting my East Village apartment in 1982, added to the fumes I'd already inhaled while painting my Washington, DC, apartment ten years earlier. How bad are latex fumes?

Maybe I got it because I dated Michael for five years, waiting, waiting, waiting for him to be ready to take the next big, scary step—*live together.*

I got it because I didn't have enough orgasms. That's what one doctor said.

I got it because I loved cats but never had one of my own.

I got it because I loved to sing and dance but didn't do either nearly enough.

Breasts are symbols of nurturing. Maybe I didn't give enough. Or get enough.

I got it because for years I was ashamed of my teeny breasts.

Did I get it as some kind of cosmic retribution for lying—for wearing huge falsies, size *A* cup, when, for example, I played Julia in Noel Coward's *Fallen Angels*?

I got it because in graduate school at Berkeley, balanced person that I was, I scarfed down a bag of cookies—either chocolate chip or peanut butter—oozing with sugar and trans fats, five nights a week.

I got it because of all the feelings I swallowed along with

those yummy cookies. I was only studying engineering because I thought it would help me get a better job—an English major trying to be practical.

Perhaps I got it because, when I was twenty-two, I smoked a joint someone had laced with LSD.

Or was it because in 1979, I tripped while hiking in the Adirondacks and fell on my breasts?

Maybe I got it because my mother was depressed—poor thing—while I was in her womb. My father was away, fighting the Japanese in the Pacific. Plus, she had to go live with her know-it-all mother-in-law.

Maybe I got it because one night when I was five, my parents wouldn't let me stay up to see *The Ed Sullivan Show* and I had, I'm told, an ear-shattering fit, or because when I ran away from home that night—to the end of the block—the blue-black quiet scared the bejesus out of me, and I had a comparable fit all the way home.

I wonder if I got it because whenever I did the shoulder stand in yoga, my breasts were upside down? That's it! I'm sure that's it! And I got it in my left breast because I always sleep on my right side!

Phew, what a relief to figure it out.

3 ꙮ

From Finding Fault to Finding Violets

April 11, 1992

Dear Ms. Nape,

I really could have used a session with you today. This talented chiropractor I've been going to for years refuses to see me now that I've had breast cancer.

But what do you care? You won't see me either. Nope, you refuse to see me less frequently than once a week, and you won't lower your $100 counseling fee.

One would think you'd be more flexible since your sessions aren't covered by health insurance. One would think you'd be more flexible since you are a breast cancer survivor too, as well as a psychotherapist who specializes in cancer survivors. You must know that many of us are already spending a lot of non-reimbursable money on our <u>physical</u> health.

I have already told you that my two sessions with you were the most helpful I have had with any counselor since I was diag-

nosed. But why do I bother repeating this since you are obviously immune to flattery as well as guilt?

You said to focus on solutions. Right, solutions. How could I afford you? By not paying my rent and going homeless. That would work. But it could get messy. I could get messy and smelly, and then I might lose my clerking job. And where would I put all my stuff?

Hey, I know. I can stand outside Memorial Sloan-Kettering and pimp for you. "Want a great therapist? She'll see you every single week, only $100 a session!" I'll find you ten new patients a week, you'll give me ten percent commission and, bingo, I can have my sessions! What do you think? You'd get richer and richer! Not that you're in it for the money.

Sincerely,

I mailed it.

I didn't realize I was angry after my mastectomy—angry at losing a breast, angry at getting cancer, angry that I might get it again, and angry that I couldn't get back on track as an actress. I didn't express this anger to my friends and family, who were so solicitous of me, and I never screamed or kicked or punched anything when I was with my regular therapist, Harriet, or when I was alone. I think I was too overwhelmed with fear—fear of my body, of more cancer and of my thoughts. Could that former surgeon Bernie Siegel be right? Did the body respond to thoughts, as he claimed in *Love, Medicine and Miracles*? Could negative thoughts cause more disease?

I knew I felt sad. I cried a lot. I never knew when the tears would come—when I woke up, tried to fall asleep, while waiting for the cross-town bus at Eighty-sixth Street? One morning a slight white-haired woman, her head shaking slightly from side to side, approached the bus shelter tiny step by tiny step, steadying herself with a cane. I lost it when she stopped, looked around with glazed eyes and smiled as if in thankful prayer for all the time given her.

But *angry* about getting cancer? I wouldn't have said I felt angry about it.

I'm sure it would have been very helpful to express my anger in private writing, in my journal, but angry words simply wouldn't come out—except in letters. I seemed to encounter person after person, most of whom I hardly knew, who infuriated me, and I felt compelled to communicate my displeasure by snail mail.

There was the macrobiotic doctor in Rochester, across New York State on the shore of Lake Ontario.

April 18, 1992

Dear Dr. McCann,

I am not paying your $50 fee for the follow-up phone consult I had scheduled with you for yesterday. I called your office four times to cancel and each time your phone was busy. Then you called at 1:00, the time of my appointment, and accused me of lying about my efforts to cancel. What can I say, doc? It's your word against mine.

You asked why I wanted to cancel and I have to admit, I did lie here, making the lame excuse that I had a scheduling conflict. I somehow managed to pick up the phone, didn't I? I do apologize. It is never good to lie, don't you agree? The truth: I wanted to cancel because, while you said on the phone a few weeks ago, before I took the six-hour train ride to your office in Rochester, that you had had "experience" helping cancer survivors follow a macrobiotic diet and lifestyle, when I saw you, you admitted that actually you had worked with only one survivor, a personal friend. I suppose this might qualify as "experience"— I wouldn't accuse you of lying—but it is considerably skimpier than I'd hoped. Considerably.

Sincerely,

Then there was the health food restaurant.

April 26, 1992

Dear Burdock Root,

You have just lost a customer.
The sign on your window says you are "macrobiotic." But to-day I learned from one of your waitresses that you use margarine and sugar in cooking and a microwave to heat food. If I wanted practices like these, I'd go to McDonald's. I and others with health concerns have been frequenting your restaurant because we have been under the impression it is "macrobiotic." We have been rely-ing on your integrity.
Get yourself a macrobiotic consultant and smell the miso!

Sincerely,

Even people who had no connection with health received angry missives, like the tenant two floors down, on the first floor, of my apartment building.

April 27, 1992

Dear Bark Avenue Boutique,

I am calling the police on Friday unless you cease and desist! I have asked you nicely three times, once in a lovely British accent, to stop blasting your radio out your air shaft window and to close this window when your dogs are barking. Apparently you find it

incomprehensible that the rest of us tenants with air shaft win-
dows don't like being serenaded by country western music and
the vocal protests of poodles and terriers as you de-fur them.

FYI, another tenant, who shall remain nameless, said she—
or he—was going to start throwing raw eggs and tomatoes at
your window, or rather through it. Naturally, I objected, "That
would be so tasteless!" Well, let's hope she—or he—won't be
driven to it.

Sincerely,

These are just a few of my written rants. I mailed them
all. The Bark Avenue proprietor didn't leash in her ways, so I
did call the police. The music and barks continued. One day,
tomatoes in one hand, eggs in the other, both arms cocked, I
imagined myself the scrappy Mrs. Peachum, the eighteenth-
century London underworld character I once played in *The
Beggar's Opera.* But I lowered my arms and made an omelet
instead. I couldn't further traumatize the poor pooches.

My therapist totally endorsed my letter writing. "Why
should you put up with any of them!" Harriet declared. A
small woman with a big mind and an even bigger heart, she
supported my dispatches as "expressions of righteous indigna-
tion" and "healthy self-assertion." In retrospect, I'm sure she
realized that these people served as catalysts to un-dam the
flood of anger inside me.

Still, surely none of my letter recipients were innocent.
None of them even bothered to write me back or call. A few
"sorry"s would have been nice—but unnecessary. I began to
think of myself as a lieutenant of Kali, the dark Hindu goddess with the lolling, bloodthirsty tongue, four arms and a
string of human skulls around her neck. Kali, divine in her
wrath, was intent on slaying evil everywhere.

May 12, 1992

Dear Dr. Spencer,

I am not sending you the $200 balance on your $400 fee. Okay, you are the most knowledgeable cancer expert I have found to date, and you did send me a detailed analysis of my health and the most comprehensive program for preventing more cancer I have ever seen—from pancreas supplements to trampoline jumping. I am grateful.

But this morning I learned that you have yet to return the numerous phone calls from my friend Tish. Could you possibly be smiling as you think of your deposit of Tish's check of $400 US, which is supposed to entitle her to phone consults with you for at least a year? Are you laughing, you son of a bitch, as you press the play button on your answering machine, and listen to Tish, lying in agony in her bed, pleading day after day after day for your advice?

Don't bother feigning concern for us anymore. We wouldn't call you again if our lives depended on it.

You might get a call from our lawyer, though. You are not immune to the consequences of fraud up there in Canada.

Sincerely,

Not that we could afford a lawyer, but possibly the threat swayed Dr. Spencer to consider forswearing his "Hypocritic Oath" in favor of the Hippocratic one.

I was very worried about Tish, but then she called a few days later to say she'd found someone in New Jersey to help her.

A VISIT WITH MY FRIEND JEAN finally helped me. I mentioned my letter-writing campaign in a phone call. "Putting a lot of energy into it, aren't you?" she commented. "Why don't you come up for the weekend?"

"I'm hanging up to pack!"

Jean lived in a bucolic spot in northwest Connecticut, a two-hour bus ride from New York, far from the city noise, Memorial Sloan-Kettering and my computer, now stuffed with nasty letters. I hadn't seen nearly enough of my old friend over the past twenty-eight years. We'd both moved around too much. She was like a treasured bottle of black-berry brandy I'd savor sips of whenever possible—not that anyone could bottle Jean.

She met me at the one-room bus station in Southbury, Connecticut, on a cool afternoon in late May, and drove us in her sputtering gray Ford van further north, through rounded hills lush with trees, by sparkling lakes and rushing streams, to Washington Depot. Past the village green, we climbed a narrow, winding road for about a mile to a small white cape. Jean had her own outdoor staircase to the two small rooms she rented on the second floor.

She turned off the ignition just as I was winding up a fury-filled account of Dr. Spencer. "I told that despicable creep off in words he won't forget!"

Jean stared out the windshield but I could see she was pull-ing her closed lips tightly across her teeth. I sighed, comforted by her obvious display of empathetic anger.

She was angry alright. Turning toward me and looking deep into my eyes, she said sternly, "You won't forget either. You're a broken record with all those letters."

"Jean!"

She opened her car door. "Come on. We need salad." She bounded to the backyard of the house in her tan jersey and brown cotton drawstring pants, with her bushy, blonde mane trailing behind, glowing white in the lingering light. I fol-lowed at a walk, still in shock at her unminced words, but giggling too. She's a six-foot forest nymph, I thought, and though her face and hands might be a bit more weathered since we first met at that boarding house near the University of Colorado, her exuberance is still a fast-forward sunrise.

I had seen the back of the house on previous visits—a faded patch of dried out weeds was what I remembered. But today it was a verdant tangle of spring growth. With her large, strong hands, Jean uprooted clumps of delicate low-lying stems covered with tiny green leaves and white flowers. She gave me some and started eating. "Chickweed. Loaded with vitamins and minerals."

"You don't wash it first?" Jean made a disparaging smirk and continued eating, so I questioned no more and nibbled. It had a refreshing taste—similar to corn but slightly edgy.

Jean picked something else. "Lamb's-quarters. Lots of beta-carotene." It reminded me of spinach.

Next she picked the leaves of something I actually recognized—that nemesis of US lawns, the lowly dandelion.

"Dandelion leaves?" I gasped.

"Good for the liver," she explained between chews. The leaves tasted bitter, but I smiled at finally feeling thankful to the plant.

Last, my friend directed me to a robust patch of violets. "Pick the flowers *and* leaves. Good for the heart." It didn't seem right to eat the darling little purple flowers, but I did as instructed. I tried to swallow them whole, imagining that they could somehow stay alive inside me.

I had never foraged before. The wild abundance and generosity surrounding me left me speechless, as did my ignorance. I would have walked right by, if not trampled, all of it.

"What do you want to do for dinner?" Jean asked.

"I don't know."

"How about a rare cheeseburger, french fries and a tall beer?"

I laughed at her eclectic palate. None of this all-American fare was part of my current cautious, organic, vegetarian diet. "My treat. I'm sure there'll be something I can eat."

So the weekend went, with Jean always ten steps ahead of me. We didn't speak of my nasty letters again.

My versatile friend, formerly a twin engine pilot and glider plane instructor, was currently supporting herself by tending the gardens of rich weekenders from New York. On Saturday, I accompanied her to one of her jobs, down a mile-long dirt driveway to an old, well-preserved white clapboard farmhouse surrounded by gently sloping fields of long grass—future hay, Jean informed me.

Since I could barely tell a hosta from a holly, definitely not a spade from a trowel, I settled at the base of an old maple tree. Jean's long, lean body moved with the grace and focus of a ballet dancer through the flower beds, pulling weeds, pruning, watering, sprinkling handfuls of a turquoise granulated fertilizer like fairy dust. I watched, inhaling the perfume of apple blossoms from a nearby tree, the tangy smell of freshly mowed grass, the potpourri of scents from the yellow, orange and white, pink, purple and lavender and also very green gardens. Squirrels played tag across the lawn, birds sang their repertoires, bees hummed among the flowers. Life celebrated life.

Sunday morning Jean and I took a walk through the woods behind her apartment to a stream as wide as Broadway. We sat on rocks and let ourselves be lulled by the gurgling water, the darkness bubbling into white. On our way back, we lunched on garlic leaves and garlic mustard, more chickweed, sheep sorrel—sour—and many more violets—sweet.

Heading home on the bus, I felt infused with fresh air, sunshine, rushing water, leaves, weeds and flowers. Thank you, dear Jean, string bean, evergreen, May Queen, genie Jeannie of the greens.

I didn't write any more nasty letters. More people annoyed me. My decency-challenged landlord, for example, refused to allow me to sublet my apartment, so I couldn't afford to rent a cabin near Jean for the summer. But after my weekend with her, it seemed a waste of time to tell off the jerk in a letter. I let out a few expletives about him at one of my sessions with Harriet, and that was the end of it. At the same time, I began to voice a few expletives about cancer with Harriet. But I didn't feel this urge very often. To be angry about anything seemed a waste of time.

Somehow I heard of a woman who led edible weed walks in Central Park. Less than a mile from my apartment I ate garlic mustard, lamb's-quarters, wild garlic and lots of violets—taking a huge leap of faith that none of the thousands of dogs in the city had peed on any of it. Jean came to visit one weekend and we foraged in the park together. By September, I was foraging on my own. Near the park wall at Central Park West and Seventy-ninth Street, I feasted on a lush swath of violets. All the delicate flowers had shriveled long ago, but the heart-shaped leaves, still deep green, tasted fresh, vibrant. Sitting in my windowless kitchen weeks later, I smiled just thinking about the wild greenness of the leaves and of Jean, and of me too.

4 ൲

Balance

I COULD HAVE KEPT MY LEFT BREAST. BUT I CON-
sulted with several doctors in New York, and, of those whose
opinion I respected, all recommended a mastectomy instead
of a lumpectomy and radiation because of the aggressive nature of my cancer cells. Oh, they also thought a mastectomy
the better alternative in my case because of the small size—
"*very* small size" one doctor felt compelled to emphasize—of
my breast.

I considered having my left chest re-amplified afterwards.
The first plastic surgeon I consulted took a quick look at me
and said with a chuckle, "Why bother, Miss Cummings? Let's
face it, men aren't attracted to you for your breasts." Speak for
yourself, buddy, I thought to respond the moment he left the
exam room, and, by the way, you might want to cut those hairs
protruding from your nose.

A more sensitive plastic surgeon told me it would be a rather simple procedure to have a saline implant inserted, unless

I wanted the "TRAM flap," which would entail his tunneling some of my abdominal skin, fat and muscle under my skin to form a breast. The TRAM flap would be far superior to the implant, he explained enthusiastically, because not only would I have feeling in my new breast but also I'd get a tummy tuck!

I hemmed and hawed about my choices for days. My chest would look more normal with an implant, at least with my clothes on. Two breasts were certainly de rigueur, despite asymmetry being admired in countless other areas of human interest from hairstyles to multimillion dollar paintings. Would I have to do more or fewer sit-ups with a TRAM flap?

My brother, Peter, who I know loves me very much, was calling frequently from his home in Santa Fe during this time. One night he asked, "Are you sure you want to go with the mastectomy?"

"Of course. The doctors said I should. A lumpectomy is more iffy."

"But what about the quality of your life?"

What was Peter thinking? The volume of my voice doubled. "I'm more sure of *living* with a mastectomy!"

"I mean, wouldn't it be better to live as long as you can with both your breasts than to live without one?"

"You've got to be kidding!" He was obviously convinced that no man would want me unless I had the conventional pair of breasts, and further, that my life wouldn't be worth living without a man! How could he, of all people, think this way? His life centered on the unconventional: his sometimes whimsical, sometimes iconic paintings and sculptures, the highly original voice of his dense poems, his wonderfully idiosyncratic friends. But, I had to admit, at over six feet, slim and strong, with thick, wavy salt-and-pepper hair and eyes that drifted from brown to green, he was one conventionally handsome dude at forty-nine, who could pass for a cousin of Paul

Newman. And, still single, he only dated conventionally gorgeous women, who, I was sure, all sported two breasts.

"Maybe you could do reconstruction. A friend out here says it can look pretty natural."

I hadn't had a date for several years, since my now good friend Michael and I had stopped being *intimes*, and I longed for a man. The prospect of never dating again seemed unbearably grim. But my brother's words galvanized my decision. "I'm not having a saline implant—anything foreign—in my body just so some man will find me physically acceptable!"

"I didn't mean—"

"I'm sure I would do reconstruction if I were big-breasted. My sense of balance would be off. But my sense of balance will be virtually the same."

A WEEK BEFORE MY MASTECTOMY, IN late March 1992, I saw my surgeon in her office at Memorial Sloan-Kettering. "The operation will take less than two hours," she said cheerily.

My left breast still felt sore below the nipple from the biopsy. Will it be that easy to remove this dear, if diseased, part of me? I wanted to run the twenty blocks north to my apartment, burrow under my fluffy rose pink comforter and sleep away the whole cancer nightmare.

My face must have reflected my anguish. "Don't worry," Dr. S consoled. "You will just be prepubescent on your left side."

Will be? She'd seen my barely AA breasts. I guess she couldn't think of anything else to say.

She lopped off my left breast in a mere hour and twenty-nine minutes.

Two days later, bandaged and glowing with relief that the cancer was out of me, I learned that my brother wasn't the only one to worry about my asymmetry. I was packing my bag to leave the hospital when a nurse I'd never seen before rushed into my semiprivate room. My roommate, who had had a mastectomy the day before, was down the hall, visiting yet another breast cancer patient. "No one gave you one yet!" the matronly woman shrieked, patting a hand on her chest to calm herself. She thrust her other hand toward me, dangling what I was about to learn was a special white mastectomy bra stuffed with lamb's wool on the left side. "Take it home, and promise me you'll get a silicone breast form as soon as you can."

"Thank you." I was touched by her concern. And I wasn't in the mood to present what by now had become almost a political position: I will go braless, obviously one-breasted. I'll say, "This is what one-breasted looks like," a variation of Gloria Steinem's "This is what fifty looks like."

My surgeon removed the bandage a week later, and, standing before my bedroom mirror that night, I was stunned. I'd been expecting to see a neat circular spot, as if Dr. S could have suctioned my breast out of my nipple. I hadn't considered this—a reddish band of varying width that extended from my left armpit to my sternum, with my left ribs as prominent as they'd been when I was ten. My left chest was hideous, my asymmetry freakish. I resolved immediately *not* to flaunt my one-breastedness. People would give me pitying stares. Men would run the other way. And I was an actress. What director would choose an obviously one-breasted woman over a two-breasted one?

LUCKILY, THERE WERE NO OTHER CUSTOMERS in the tiny boutique on the Upper West Side, which was stuffed floor to ceiling with plastic drawers and wooden cupboards full of lingerie. The woman behind the glass counter, chic in her peach

Donna Karan suit, with her gray hair in a classic chignon, gave me a welcoming smile. I leaned a forearm on the counter and let slither out the side of my mouth, "I need a silicone breast form—small as they come."

"Absolutely!" She walked crisply to a back room and returned with a shiny white box. Handing me the floppy flesh-colored slab, she brushed it lightly as if admiring the latest fashion trend.

I touched the top of the gel-filled prosthesis gingerly with my fingertips. It did feel remarkably reminiscent of my former breast. Of course, I thought, one cat claw could deconstruct it into a gooey mess.

Bernice—we were already on a first-name basis—picked up a satiny, admirably roomy beige bra from the counter and demonstrated how she could sew special envelopes into the left side of my bras to hold the form in place. I raced home and brought her a few of my white plain-Jane AAs.

Two days later, sporting my new breast system underneath a brand-new red pants suit, I strutted out of her shop. I felt très à la mode on that fresh May morning, parading down Broadway—a bit like Auntie Mame, a character I was born to play, after she'd conquered some trivial adversity. But I'd gone less than a block when the bra started to ride up. What was I thinking? My bras had always ridden up. If two barely AA breasts couldn't keep a bra down, how could one?

A few days later, a woman in the locker room at my gym whipped a silicone breast off her left chest and showed me the Velcro strip attached to the breast form, as well as the mate strip glued across her chest. "I just love it!" she raved. "I can even wear it under my swimming suit!"

I was happy the clever get-up worked for her. But for myself, the prospect of having a detachable breast made me feel like Raggedy Ann, pieced together with ersatz this and that.

Besides, putting glue on my chest was out of the question. I didn't even want to rub in Vitamin E oil, which would have helped heal my scar, because I was terrified that any stimulation to the area might promote the growth of cancer cells.

I couldn't have worn a Velcroed breast anyway. One day my mail included a catalogue from a Florida company offering all kinds of breast supports, diminishers and enhancers, and on impulse I called to inquire about a Velcro form. The cost was $395, close to my rent at the time, and, besides, the smallest available form was out of my league—an A.

So there I was with my scar, braless most of the time. I would wear layered or very loose tops to camouflage the flatness on the left side of my chest—and the only slightly raised right side. I tried thinking of myself as one of the Amazons, those mythic Greek warrior women who each cut off a breast in order to shoot arrows more easily. But I didn't have the slightest impulse to take up archery, and in my case a breast wouldn't have been in the way at all.

After three months or so, I did begin to touch my left side lightly, feeling my heart beat closer beneath my hand, feeling my ribs more directly. At some point during the summer, I promised myself I would look at my chest in my bedroom mirror every morning. It was shocking every time. I seemed so ugly, so far, far away from normal.

By late fall, I must have become somewhat more used to my new normal. One day, wandering around the Metropolitan Museum of Art with no conscious agenda, I came upon Toulouse-Lautrec's lithograph *Jane Avril*. A strong, gray-black hand holds the thick gray-black neck of a viol, which extends diagonally from the bottom center of the poster to the upper right. This diagonal is offset by another one—the high-kicking, black-stockinged leg of Jane Avril, a cancan dancer, in her full orange skirt. The simple bold lines and colors created a lively balance *without* symmetry. Did my new body have a lively balance too?

I rushed home to view the entire front of my body in my mirror. I considered my large features primarily background—the long and fairly unremarkable face (except for the time I landed the role of a woman supposedly chosen from an infomercial audience, and I was glamorized with Dr. F.'s Face Care Products); the wild, kinky hair; the hourglass figure, with considerably more hours below the waist than above; the long legs accented by size ten feet.

That day I was interested in the finer details. On my left side, I noted the now whitish diagonal scar on my chest; a flesh-colored scar above my eye, thanks to a tumble from my first two-wheeler; a large brown freckle in the middle of my thigh; and two white vertical scars of forgotten origin on my shin. On the right side were only my understated breast and a long white vertical scar on the shin, a souvenir from a hike years earlier on the Olympic Peninsula near Seattle.

My arms were hanging down at my sides, with the hands slightly curved, the index and pinky fingers slightly raised. Was I balanced? Not quite. But then I extended my right arm horizontally and bent it up at the elbow. *Voilà*, a dynamic work of art—maybe not Metropolitan material, definitely not a *Playboy* centerfold, but, well, perhaps a neo-Paul Klee with whimsical hieroglyphics. I was delighted.

But then, celebrating my triumph with a cup of peach tea, my mood suddenly crashed. Who would ever share my new appreciation of my body? The rest of the world expected—men would accept nothing less than, according to my brother—two symmetrical breasts. I began to feel a kinship with Toulouse-Lautrec: his legs were stunted, and he was considered deformed too. I remembered that he had frequented places where he had felt accepted—the brothels, cabarets, music halls and theaters of late nineteenth-century Paris. Where could I go?

One cold still day in early December, I had to meet a friend on Broadway and decided to walk there through Central Park. Shortly after entering the quasi-sylvan refuge at East Seventy-ninth Street, my eyes were drawn to a tree with craggy bark whose trunk curved gracefully toward the ground and then bounded up to the sky. I found its shape beautiful. Would I feel this way about every tree I looked at in the park, I wondered, or would some of them seem ugly?

I considered hundreds of deciduous trees. They had already lost most of their leaves so, unlike the evergreens, their dark trunks and branches were clearly displayed against the light-gray sky. There was a tree with enormous burls on its trunk, one with a trunk coiled like a spastic corkscrew, another with a trunk about four feet in diameter and spindly branches. Another tree couldn't decide which way to grow. Its various branches arched downward, stretched out diagonally and horizontally, arched upwards and shot straight up. Another tree had a gash at least seven feet long up its trunk. Many trees had cut limbs. The branches on the north side of one had all been sawed off long ago, leaving holes like deep-set eyes. On the bank of the lake near West Seventy-second Street, a tree trunk had snapped. The upper half, still partially attached to the lower, had fallen into the lake, and along the portion still above water, a line of young sprigs reached toward the sky.

Before exiting the park at West Eighty-first, I leaned against the smooth bark of a tree whose branches wove intricately under, over and around each other like a giant nest. None of the trees I was attracted to in the park was symmetrical, I realized.

They were all asymmetrical in wonderfully different ways. I'd found every one of them beautiful. Surely I wasn't the only person to notice this—that the unique eccentricities of trees, including their injuries, didn't detract from but rather contributed to, were integral to, were at the very core of their beauty.

5 ॐ

If I'd Only Kept Dancing

I FELT BEAUTIFUL AT THE DANCES EVERY OTHER SAT-
urday night all summer long when I was a teenager. On the
shore of usually tranquil Little Moose Lake in the Adirondack
Mountains, the large community room above the boathouse
would be boisterous with happy conversation and laughter.
In colorful dresses, and khaki pants and pastel sports jackets,
the grownups and we teenagers—all people who summered
in houses around the lake—would sashay around the room
to Lester Lanin's gay "Just One of Those Things" and "I Love
Paris." His band put out one hot record after another in the
latter half of the 1950s.

I would stand with my girlfriend Callie by one of the open
windows, swaying to the music, often in my favorite dress, a
strapless blue paisley cotton with navy blue zigzag piping along
the top and at the waist. The dress had been my mother's,
which still astounds me since she was five foot two, and I was
already taller by age thirteen. Maybe it fit me because Ma had

filled the bodice outward with her Bs, while I, barely AAA back then, stretched it upward with my height. I didn't fill even a third of my padded white strapless bra. Somehow neither the bra nor the dress ever fell down.

The cool Adirondack mountain air would blow through the spruces, across Little Moose and over my shoulders until the magic moment when one of the teenage boys would ask me to dance. I had a crush—totally unrequited—on tall, blond, blue-eyed Johnny Dyett. Johnny and I would two-step together, smooth as soft butter spreads, over the creaky floor. I felt beautiful all over.

If I'd only kept dancing. In the fall, I was sent off to an all-girls boarding school in Massachusetts. Northampton School for Girls did arrange the occasional "mixer" with an all-boys boarding school, but these brief encounters were about gyrating to Chubby Checker and Dion, and, wrapped around a total stranger, rocking from one foot to the other to dreamy Johnny Mathis. They were never about graceful movement. Our family moved to a different town in Westchester County, north of New York City, during my freshman year, and I never met anyone—usually a prerequisite for dancing with someone—when I was home on vacations. Then off I went to college and later to one profession after another and, except for the rare night of gyrating and clinging, I didn't dance again until my mid-forties.

Confidence in my physical appearance first surfaced as an issue in sixth grade when Jessie Steinfeld told a gaggle of us girls on the playground that she was wearing her first bra. Her mother told her she had to, she boasted, because her breasts were so big. I had been one of the most popular girls in class until then. But, I swear, within weeks, I, with my two pimples, became of less and less interest, while Jessie, who had been shy, always a follower, and who lacked any apparent academic interests, blossomed into a confident leader, one of the most sought after by both girls and boys.

Week after week, it seemed, yet another girl would announce that she had started to wear a bra, until, by seventh grade, I begged my mother to get me one too. South we sped in our family's wood-paneled station wagon to Alexander's Department Store in White Plains, in pursuit of the bra with the longest straps and the smallest cups, padded, of course, ever made. By this time, I was the extreme on two counts—the tallest and the flattest girl in class—and I had covered the mirror above my bedroom bureau with black construction paper. My mother and father would continuously remind me to "stand up straight." Why? To flaunt my nothingness? How I envied normally endowed girlfriends, who could wear clingy tops. I limited myself to blousy ones, on the outside chance that at least undiscerning eyes would view me as vaguely proportional. In locker rooms, I undressed in the toilet stalls. My swimming suits had to have firmly formed cups because otherwise my underdevelopment would have been way overexposed. The cups were always size A or B, which was kind of fun, but I had to be careful not to brush up against anyone lest they collapse.

I wanted breasts. As soon as I got my driver's license at sixteen, I drove to Alexander's alone to buy two foam ones, an A-cup bra and also a skimpy, red V-necked cotton top. After locking the bathroom door, I rushed to put on my booty and viewed myself in the mirror from every possible angle. *Va-va-va-voom*! I was Sophia Loren's sister!

But if I walked out of the bathroom so enhanced, what would my parents say? Surely, my brother Peter would burst into hysterics. And what if I wore my A-look to one of those school mixers and got romantic with some guy? He might start feeling around and discover that he shouldn't have judged my book by my cover. I hid my contraband in the back of the top shelf of my closet, resurrecting it briefly now and then to gaze wistfully at what could have been mine but for an aberrant gene. My mother was a perfectly adequate B. My sister Nancy was a C.

Breasts were sticking out everywhere in America at the time, not only on an alarming number of lucky-duck friends, but in magazines, newspapers and movies and on TV. Men were going gaga over Sophia and Marilyn, Jayne and Liz. My father, a successful, globetrotting advertising executive, who knew the importance of the image of a product to the marketing of it, must have worried that I'd be a tough sell in this voluptuous environment. One evening when I was home for winter break during my freshman year at Northwestern University, he asked if I wanted to get breast augmentation implants. "No!" I snapped and ran to my bedroom. Breast implants? My father, the most important man in my life at this point, thought I needed breast implants? Usually distant and stern, he was concerned enough about my prospects to take the time to offer me implants?

Actually, another female icon, Twiggy, the skinny, flat fashion model, was popular in the 1960s, but I knew, and I guess my father must have too, that I didn't look like this one either. My breasts fit the bill, but even at my slimmest, my derriere was at least three times Twiggy's. Besides, Twiggy seemed admired mostly by women. My brother never dated a Twiggy.

My father only mentioned his offer that one time, and through the years, I would wish I'd accepted it every time I'd see a man give me the once-over, gape at the lack of three-dimensionality of my chest and move on. I could have lured men in with the implants—until they fell in love with my irresistible personality.

But I never did get augmented. I guess the idea of someone cutting into my breasts to insert silicone or saline pads was always too repugnant, an unacceptable violation to my body and also to me as a person. My small breasts, whether I liked them or not, were an integral part of who I was, along with my hazel eyes, kinky mop, loud laugh, love of cats and consumption of chocolate as an essential food group.

I did augment them temporarily for a few auditions and roles. This arrangement worked well—I was usually chosen for fairly sexually reserved characters—except for the time I played Mistress Page in *The Merry Wives of Windsor.* The director asked why I refused to wear a costume with a very low-cut neckline. "Uh, well ... I'm ... I mean Mistress Page is prudish."

Sometimes I even enjoyed my dainty orbs—when steaming water would shower over them, when the sun or a living room fire would warm them through my clothes. I liked the way pajamas and well-worn sweatshirts brushed over them like feathers. Now and then I liked to caress them. Occasionally I would massage them with oil.

My boyfriends, few though they were, never ridiculed my minimalist breasts. One fellow called them "very sweet." All my lovers seemed to enjoy touching, kissing, sucking and rubbing themselves against them. I certainly enjoyed these activities. When I was thirty, Ted, my boyfriend at the time, bought me a thin, tight-fitting lavender wool sweater with a low-scooped neck, made in Paris. He said small-breasted women looked "sexy as Hell" in tight sweaters when they went braless, which he asked me to do, and I did, with him. My most recent ex, Michael, smiled whenever I paraded around my apartment or his in my black bikini panties and my one black bra—only worn on special occasions. Michael said he loved to look at me in my "black fantastics," as he called them. I was particularly flattered because he had a great eye. When he wasn't at his day job editing music and sound effects for films and videos, he was usually off shooting exquisite photographs of nature.

Still, I continued to feel primarily shame for my junior-junior-juniors until, ironically, a couple of years before the left one had to be removed. In my mid-forties, an acting coach recommended I take an improvisational dance class for actors in midtown. The women were required to wear black leotards and tights and the men, white T-shirts and black tights. These outfits left nothing to anyone's imagination. Before many a class, I would look in the mirrors that covered one wall of the studio and cringe at the sight of my flat chest.

The teacher, Loyd, middle-aged, tall and solid, looking positively dignified in his T-shirt and tights, would gesture to the pianist, and for the next two hours, the long-haired, long-fingered mellow fellow would fill the room with music—improvised adagios as we did warm-up stretches on the floor and then a seamless medley of classical, jazz and Broadway. I would prance and spin, reach, arch, dip, jump and jive, swept away by the music, inventing with it, either by myself or in spontaneous ensembles. After class, I would look in the mirror again and always see myself, all of me, including my two tiny breasts, as radiant, gorgeous, provocative even.

Dancing week after week, the joy of the improv class reached deeper and deeper inside me. The fond memory of two-stepping with Johnny kept occurring to me—the swishing of my lovely dress, Johnny humming a Lester Lanin tune in my ear as we glided across the floor of the community room. Eventually I understood that it hadn't been so much the dress or Johnny, but primarily my moving with and playing with the beautiful music that had made me feel beautiful. If I'd only kept dancing.

6 ↬

Searching for a Health Plan
I Can Swallow

Rrrrring. Rrrrring.
THE PHONE ON MY KITCHEN TABLE WAS ONLY SIX inches from my hand, but I was engrossed in *How To Fight Cancer and Win.* By this time, early July 1992, three months after my mastectomy, my burgeoning collection of paperbacks on healing was taking over a bookshelf. I was still Internet-phobic. This latest volume extolled the benefits of eating flaxseed oil mixed with cottage cheese—which I was already doing—and was loaded with accounts of people who had apparently cured themselves of all kinds of cancers by this simple snack. I was feeling safer by the word.

My answering machine kicked in. "I know you're there. Pick up if you dare." My actress friend Celestina was in one of her rhyming moods. "You want to see an origami rabbit?" She had started teaching herself the folding art earlier in the year and had already mastered a Noah's Ark of animals.

I picked up, still half-reading. "Male or female?"

"That would be R-rated origami. I'm only into G-rated."

"Too bad. Well, congrats on your eunuch."

"Thank you very much. So, what's up, hiccup?"

"Flaxseed oil cures cancer."

"Great! What's flaxseed oil?"

"Oil. From flaxseeds."

"Uh-huh."

"This book also recommends pancreatic enzyme pills."

"Pancake what?"

I ignored her attempt at humor. "The health food store must know about them. I'll call as soon as we hang up."

"Take it easy, sleazy."

"Take it easy?" I could feel the heat rushing to my skin. "I want to live, Celestina! I'll do anything not to get cancer again."

There was silence on the other end of the line. That was odd. In the five years I'd known her, since we suppressed sibilants together in a speech class for actors, Celestina had never been at a loss for words. I pictured her big brown Italian eyes growing even larger as she ran her fingers through her silky, shoulder-length blonde hair.

"Hello?"

"I just think . . . from one actress to another . . . you're being . . . a little melodramatic, don't you think? You only had an early-stage cancer. It didn't even get out of your breast. What did you call it—insight?"

"In situ. It could have killed me if it hadn't been detected!"

"I know, but. . . . "

"My body made it somehow, Celestina. I've got to change my body or it could make it again!"

"I hear you."

Celestina didn't really get it, I thought after we'd hung up, but that was totally understandable. I hoped to God she'd never have to get it. I dialed A Matter of Health. Yes, they had pancreatic enzyme pills. Yes, they'd set aside five bottles for me.

Why should Celestina get it? My surgeon didn't even get it, and she cut cancer out of women every day.

"You're cured now, Susan," Dr. S said authoritatively a few weeks after my mastectomy. She was leaning over me, running her index finger lightly along the shiny, now pinkish, flattened worm of a line across my left chest. I hadn't yet ventured to touch the scar myself, except to dab it ever so lightly with a towel after showers. The doctor's gesture made the area feel tingly.

"That's it?"

She flicked her red—extraordinarily red—hair behind both ears and stood up. "That's it."

That couldn't be it, I thought. I was sure I needed an anti-cancer nutritional regimen to keep me safe. I believed in nutritional regimens. About three years before my cancer was diagnosed, I'd had severe hypoglycemia, and I was sure my recovery from this debilitating condition was due to the super healthy diet and bottles and bottles of supplements a gifted chiropractor had prescribed.

There had to be a nutritional program that could protect me from more cancer. I had so many more things to do. I still hadn't played the spirited medium Madame Arcati in Noel Coward's *Blithe Spirit*, Auntie Mame or a number of Shakespeare, Tennessee Williams and Neil Simon women. I was still searching for my spiritual path. I still hadn't met my mate.

The same week I saw my surgeon, I learned of an even more compelling reason to stay alive. My therapist Harriet and I were talking in the living room of her apartment on West Eighty-seventh across the street from Central Park when suddenly it was as if I were in rehearsal for a play at the point when you effortlessly become the character, when the character moves you.

Without the slightest pause in conversation, I started talking as an effervescent five-year-old.

Harriet welcomed my regressed self immediately, calling her "Susie." When Susie asked if she could draw, Harriet pulled a big white pad and a box of crayons from a bookcase, and we both settled on her orange and brown Oriental rug. Harriet watched like a doting mother as Susie outlined and then filled in various abstract shapes.

"This is very interesting, very pretty," Harriet said. Susie giggled with pride. She would have liked to have continued drawing all day, but at some point Harriet said, "We have to stop now. We can draw again next week."

"Okay," Susie said easily.

Susie receded immediately as I got up from the floor, and a stunned forty-seven-year-old me hugged Harriet good-bye. "I don't know what just happened, but I'm so happy!"

"Me, too!" Harriet grinned. She held my hand as we walked to the door. "Do you feel okay to leave? I have another client coming."

"I feel great, a little weird but great." We both laughed.

"Be gentle with yourself today. Call if you want to talk."

I crossed the street slowly and sat on the first bench I saw in the park. Was I cracking up? I recognized Susie as a part of me, although I couldn't remember ever being as happy—completely happy—as she apparently was. She unnerved me, but still I hoped she would appear again. She seemed to know only joy and love and trust.

Harriet called that night to say she thought Susie represented a "mild psychic dissociation," totally understandable, she reassured me, in light of the trauma of having had cancer.

I wasn't versed in psych-speak. "You mean maybe I've been so afraid of dying that my soul insisted I remember the wonder of life through Susie?"

"Maybe."

"You think maybe my acting background might have helped me find the vehicle of a five-year-old?"

"Maybe." Harriet didn't think it possible to know all the answers in life, or advisable to try. To experience life was the important thing to her.

Susie would appear many times during my search for a health plan. Harriet supported my decision not to worry that her appearance might indicate I was losing my mind. I let myself enjoy "seeing" her, or perhaps more accurately "being" her. She was precious. She found every second of life precious.

I continued reading health books. One described over a hundred alternative cancer prevention programs, using terms like "tumor complement factor," "T-lymphocytes," "proteolytic enzymes" and "Essiac." Help! Despite my Masters in engineering, I was still basically an English major. I needed someone who could sift through all this confusion. The brilliant Dr. Spencer from Canada, whom I had discovered back in April, was out of the question since he had behaved so abominably with my friend Tish.

In early October, I went to the New York Open Center, an eclectic holistic learning center downtown in Soho, to hear a twenty-seven-year-old colon cancer survivor talk about the dietary program she was following. The rosy-cheeked speaker looked as fresh as the carrots, celery stalks and apples she was feeding into her gleaming Champion juicer. Her daily regimen, developed by the German, Dr. Max Gerson, included supplements, a cup of fresh juice eight times a day and two coffee enemas. My mind did somersaults, my relevant sphincter muscle clamped at the prospect of such below-the-belt caffeine rushes. Surely I'd never sleep again. And, together with that juicing schedule, when would I have time for anything else?

I didn't realize it then, but I would have a number of criteria for my health regimen, and effort would be one of them. My plan couldn't require too much of me, or too little.

"Fascinating!" a woman commented to me in the hallway after the lecture. Her blue eyes bulged with excitement as she sipped her Dixie cup of organic juice. "But I can't imagine doing all those enemas and the juicing." Her short auburn curls bobbed as she shook her head.

We continued to talk for over an hour. With her bouncy personality, I never would have guessed Lori to be two years older than I. She had come to the lecture because she was suffering from enormous and painful uterine fibroids, which every conventional doctor she'd consulted had insisted be removed surgically, along with her uterus. She rejected this option. She thought the fibroids, which had a virtually zero chance of becoming cancerous, might be shrunk by a nutritional program strong enough to prevent cancer. I couldn't follow her logic, but didn't challenge her.

"I love alternative medicine, don't you?" she gushed. "It's so positive!"

"Yes!" I agreed.

IN BETWEEN OUR PART-TIME JOBS—Lori helped her mother sell houses in Nassau County on Long Island, while I continued my lofty clerical functions at the gastroenterologist's—we launched a joint campaign to find our perfect health programs. Lori, a finance major in college, knew even less about science and medicine than I did, and she agreed that our primary goal was to find some kind of a healer we could trust.

I was confident we'd find one. We lived in New York, where the Yellow Pages were over two inches thick. Also, I was my father's daughter. Granted, this was a mixed blessing. He had criticized me constantly for years—my hair was too wild, my knapsack was too unfeminine to attract a man, my earnings were laughable. Seeing him often left me feeling limp for days. He only came once to my cozy, shower-in-the-kitchen one-bedroom walk-up on East Tenth Street, and refused to visit when I moved to a slightly larger shower-in-the-kitchen one-bedroom walk-up on East Eighty-second. My semi-Bohemian ways made him uncomfortable. He was comfortable with daughter number one—stylish, all business Nancy, who had followed him into advertising. She successfully juggled being an executive, wife and mother, and lived in an antique-appointed, two-bedroom, two-and-a-half-bath co-op in a building sentineled by doormen on the Upper West Side.

Still, Daddy could be kind, generous and also funny. He did come to some of my shows. And I admired his sharp mind, aptitude for business and drive. A transplant to New York from a small town in Illinois, he became chief executive officer of what was then one of the largest advertising agencies in the United States. He was probably my most important role model for working hard at a seemingly impossible goal until it was achieved. Surely, I could find a healer.

Lori and I looked for over a year, combing through health books and newsletters, attending at least one health-related lecture or conference a week, contacting nonprofit health groups, friends of friends, friends of friends of friends. Our researching sometimes gave me the high I remembered from ferreting out information as a young reporter for *The Northern Virginia Sun*. We never considered seeing anyone unless he or she had been highly recommended by at least one respected source.

Despite our best efforts at being discriminating, however, we saw and rejected a slew of healers, saying bye-bye to a pile of money in the process. They were unacceptable for all kinds of reasons. Some turned out to be flagrant con artists. When I asked Dr. Stevens, MD, *why* he thought I needed all of the pills on his two-page list, as well as three different herbal drinks and high doses of vitamins intravenously, he responded with a wry smile, "Why not do everything you can?" He then ushered me down the hall of his multi-roomed suite in Tarrytown, New York, to his store, which ever so helpfully sold everything he recommended. A young associate tagged along, eager to administer the drips. I told him I'd get back to him.

Dr. Rabinowicz, MD, sat across from me at his large leather-topped wooden desk in one of the many rooms in his suite on Lexington Avenue. "Anything wrong except the breast cancer history?" the short, wiry man asked as he glanced at the first page, only, of the five-page patient information form I'd just spent half an hour filling out.

"That's all," I said.

"Tell me everything," he coaxed in his eastern European accent. "One-stop shopping. Any depression in the family?"

"My brother." Pete had had to cope with manic depression and the nasty side effects of the pills to control it for almost thirty years.

"So! It's genetic!" His face lit up like a child's at Cirque de Soleil. "You've got to fight it! Fight it! Zoloft!"

"Thank you, anyway."

"In tiny amounts, there is absolutely nothing to worry about," he persisted. He leaned across his desk. "And by the way, if you need any help with hair loss, I have the only formula in the world that works."

I ran a hand through what I remembered to be a full crop of hair. It was still there.

He was a colorful rascal, I thought when I was back on the sidewalk. Maybe I'll use him someday to prepare for a role.

Some healers seemed to have competent health programs, but they disappeared. I went to Dr. Loo in Chinatown after a friend told me her herbs had shrunk the brain tumor of someone he knew to the size of a pea. At my first appointment, Dr. Loo felt my wrist pulses, asked a few questions through her receptionist-translator, and fifteen minutes later presented me with two white plastic bottles filled with powdered herbs. I was to take two dainty spoonfuls with water twice a day. I felt really safe from cancer for the first time.

But I never saw Dr. Loo again. On my second and third visits, her brother read my pulses. Dr. Loo was "in Hong Kong working," and then "on vacation," the receptionist-translator explained. Excuse me, but it was Dr. Loo's diplomas, not her brother's, that covered one wall of her tidy, walk-in closet of an office.

A cancer information center referred me to Jacob, a brilliant PhD biochemist near Philadelphia. He had written his thesis on why specific foods, from carrots to hijiki seaweed, were anticarcinogenic. Sitting in Jacob's spare, bare-walled office, I felt safe again. He approved of my diet, except for my occasional bagel.

"I can't give them up," I pleaded. "I might have an anxiety attack, lose my identity."

On my second visit, after my blood analyses came back, Jacob advised that to increase my "killer cells," I should take six maitake and six shitake mushroom pills a day. As soon as I returned to New York, I bought a bottle of each and started taking them. But within a week, I contracted the most itchy, burning yeast infection of my life. Help! I called and left Jacob a message. "You think it could be the mushroom pills?" He didn't return my call. I left a second message, a third. He never called back.

Other healers downright scared me. By the time I met Daryl, in Westport, Connecticut, I wasn't impressed one way or the other that he hadn't had a formal education in either medicine or science. I'd already rejected countless MDs and other licensed healers. The tall, stringy forty-something was very knowledgeable and bright, his enthusiasm for alternative healing was contagious, and I admired his warm compassion for the cancer patients who streamed into his compact colonial. He suggested ozone treatments to boost my immune system and give me more energy, among other benefits. Since I'd already read that thousands of health practitioners in Germany, including many MDs, were using this procedure, I was eagerly expectant, not at all frightened, when he injected me intravenously. A mere two hours after Daryl's first needle, I felt so invigorated, I wanted to jog again after a hiatus of twenty years. This was the most tangible physical change I'd experienced since my mastectomy.

But one day during a delightful chat with Sandra, another middle-aged cancer survivor, who was getting her ozone drip on the treatment table next to mine, Sandra whispered that Daryl was somehow keeping his unconscious elderly mother alive in a back room. Yikes! Hopefully, Daryl was engaging in this, shall we say, overly ambitious activity out of love for his mom, but my trust in alternative healing hit a wall. I couldn't stop thinking that I was in a science fiction thriller in which the police were about to crash through the front door.

Then there was Dr. Ribley. At first I felt very comfortable with this round, jolly man, whose warmth was reflected in his inviting Old World living room/office on Central Park West. A tape of Chopin's nocturnes showered the air with delicacy. Pointing to two bottles of Chinese herbal tinctures on a rosewood side table, the doctor explained, "All my cancer survivors take one mixture or the other." He would use "muscle testing," he said, to determine which tincture was more suitable for me. Now, to the uninitiated, muscle testing can seem as viable as the world's best hair growth spray, but I believed it worked because, though it still confounded me, the chiropractor who had cured me of hypoglycemia had used it to determine which supplements I needed.

Holding one of Dr. Ribley's bottles in my right hand, I extended my left arm to the side and tried to resist as he tried to push it down. If a tincture was to be beneficial, my arm would be strong enough to withstand his pushing.

My arm went down with each of the bottles.

"This has never happened before," the perplexed man said. Frowning now, he tried the bottles again and again. Beads of sweat formed on his forehead. He forced a smile. "I guess you don't need either of them."

Was neither tincture right because I was so healthy, or was I Dr. Ribley's first hopeless case?

Lori and I would check in by phone every day and meet for lunch or dinner at least once a week, usually at her studio apartment on East Ninetieth Street. With our chopsticks piled high with organic aduki beans, brown rice and alfalfa sprouts, all lathered with organic tahini sauce, we would discuss our latest information. Our friendship and camaraderie always recharged me. Plus, sitting on Lori's lush lime-green carpet always felt like a mini-vacation. Often I would imagine our mugs of organic green tea to be tall gin and tonics, which we were swilling in sun-drenched St. Lucia.

Eventually, I found others interested in following nutritional regimens at cancer support groups in New York and, by phone, across the continent. I was especially drawn to women who trusted the healing power of herbs. A "green witch" in the Catskills told me she drank copious cups of red clover tea. A woman outside Quebec gathered five herbs that she steeped for a week in gin—yum—before she boiled the mixture into a tea. I didn't consider drinking any of these herbal remedies without the counsel of some sort of professional healer. But the women, confident in and grateful for what they were doing and unbelievably generous to talk at length with me, inspired me to keep hunting.

Susie kept inspiring me too. She seemed to know where it was safe to "come out"—in my apartment, at Harriet's, in Central Park. She loved to walk, sometimes skip, along the asphalt paths in the park, awed by everything as if seeing it for the first time—three teenage girls laughing on a bench, roller-bladers, a man throwing a Frisbee to his poodle. A queen and a king lived in Belvedere Castle, high on the rocks, only no one could see them. Susie was in love with everything. She felt love from everything.

Through the months, I did come across several healers who seemed to have solid plans and who I didn't think would scare me or disappear, but I didn't think it should be necessary to wipe out my savings to save my life. One clinic in Mexico charged $4,000 a week for a minimum of three weeks. A well-respected center in New York wanted $1,800 for the first two visits.

Then my criterion of effort took center stage. A girlfriend who had been seeing a homeopath for years found out that he treated cancer survivors. She explained that homeopaths prescribe minute amounts of the appropriate "remedy" to stimulate a patient's own healing powers. That sounded empowering.

Consulting two thick, worn tomes in his stark office in the East Village, the earnest Dr. Watt asked me a number of questions I'd never considered before—"When it rains, are you more afraid of the lightning or the thunder?", "Do you like wall-to-wall carpets or area rugs?"—and then handed me an illegible prescription to be filled at Bigelow Pharmacy on Sixth Avenue. I let the first tiny white sugary pill dissolve under my tongue at the frantic corner of Sixth Avenue and Eighth Street, and within seconds, my entire insides felt as if all the anxieties they'd been holding onto for years had been washed away. This serenity lasted about an hour. Wow, I thought, wouldn't it be marvelous to feel this way all the time! But after popping the rest of the vial over the next week—without any more dramatic effects—I decided not to answer any more of the homeopath's intriguing questions and not to take any more pills smaller than Tic Tacs. Homeopathy didn't require enough of me.

A few weeks later, tending to a pot of organic brown rice simmering on my stove, I took deep, reverential breaths of its faintly nutty aroma, as if the smell alone were an elixir. On the adjacent counter, a strip of dried kombu seaweed was soaking in a large mug, turning the water's surface translucent emerald. I raised the shiny six-inch blade of my new Japanese knife and, as I had just been taught by Philip, my new macrobiotic counselor, chopped an onion into crescent moons, slowly, steadily, exactly. My eyes teared, releasing nameless sadnesses. I chopped a daikon into half moons, carrots into pyramids, butternut squash into large chunks, cutting out what I didn't want—this rottenness, that fear, that fear again, that fear again. The differences in the shapes pleased me. I sliced the now slimy kombu into squares, placed these in the bottom of a glass pot, added water and slid in the vegetables in order: onions, daikon, carrots, squash on top. Each vegetable was unique, I was learning, with its own character, requirements and gifts to offer. I added a pinch of sea salt and, when the water started to boil, turned the burner knob to low, covered the pot and sat to wait at my sturdy pine table conveniently located two feet away. The vegetal mist—earthy, sweet as early morning—filled the air, filled me. Soon I was eating a healthy as well as delicious dinner. I felt calm, safe, grateful.

But all that chopping, boiling and steaming, not to mention sautéing, pressure cooking, baking, pickling and yin-yang food combining, took hours. Macrobiotics was way too much work.

A couple of weeks later, an exotic muskiness filled my apartment as I boiled a paper packet worth of dried roots, stems, leaves, flowers and unidentifiable vegetal matter that Dr. Chen, another Chinatown herbalist, had prescribed for me. I was to boil a packet of herbs for an hour, drink the liquid, reboil the same herbs the next day, drink; boil the next packet, drink, reboil, drink; boil the next packet, drink, reboil, drink. Every time I drank a cup of the reddish-brown bittersweet liquid, I imagined I was being filled with the essence of deep forests and sunny meadows. I felt rooted, rebloomed, definitely safe.

But I was trapped at home every day by that incessant boiling.

Susie began to come out in more places—once at Celestina's forty-first birthday party in an Italian restaurant in the West Village. Luckily, all four of us were actresses, used to seeing each other take on different roles. But then she appeared in an improvisation workshop that a friend convinced me to visit one night. My improv was supposed to be about a man in a bar picking up a woman, not a five-year-old. Where would Susie show up next? My sweet "mild psychic dissociation" was out of control. I had to find a health plan!

SUSIE STOPPED APPEARING ON OCTOBER 3, 1993. Like every woman who goes for her annual mammogram, especially those of us at higher risk for malignancies, I was grateful for, but also terrorized by, my appointment at Memorial Sloan-Kettering that morning. After the technician x-rayed my right breast, I sat in the dressing cubicle waiting for the verdict. Rivulets of sweat dripped from my armpits onto the pastel green paper gown.

The technician knocked. "We have to take another shot, Miss Cummings."

They saw something! They saw something just like before!

Another X-ray. Another wait. A lot more sweat.

"Everything's fine, Miss Cummings. You can go home now."

Hooray! Provided neither I nor my surgeon during her yearly kneading of my breast finds a lump, I have another cancer-free year to live! This deserves a celebration.

On my walk back uptown, I stopped at A Matter of Health on First Avenue for a mixed vegetable juice. Actually I had stopped at this health food store for fresh juice practically every day since my mastectomy, but it seemed like a special treat today. Standing by the counter drinking, I resolved that, by God, I'd make it my full-time, not just part-time, job to find my cancer prevention program.

And don't you know, also standing near the counter was this thirty-something yuppie in a white button-down shirt, chocolate brown cords and loafers without socks. "You should skip the carrots," he advised. The blandly attractive blond tipped his cup toward me so I could see that his juice was parsley green, not orange like mine.

"Excuse me?"

"Too much sugar."

"To each, her or his own," I said lightly.

"I know it's confusing, but you're better off not juicing them." He spoke lackadaisically, as if fueled by Muzak.

Mr. Smarty Pants was obviously an idiot. "Carrots are loaded with beta carotene. Read any nutrition book."

"Don't believe everything you read."

"You're an expert?"

"No, but I know people who are." He handed me a sun-yellow business card. STEVEN SIMMS ALTERNATIVE HEALTH INFORMATION BROKER was embossed in parsley green.

There's definitely a market for such people, I thought.

"I know a brilliant guy if you're by chance looking for a cancer expert."

How could he tell? Was it the orange tinge to my skin from all the carrot juice? But I wasn't a pushover. I had criteria. "Is he into Chinese herbs?"

"No."

"Macrobiotics? Homeopathy?"

"No, no. He uses supplements, lots of supplements."

I could do supplements. "You think he's going to stick around awhile?"

"Joseph? He's more New York than Zabar's."

Hearing the name of this institution of gourmet delights, my mouth immediately salivated for its hundred percent fat cheeses, paper-thin slices of smoked salmon and buttery chocolate rugelach. More germane to the moment, the super deli had been at Eightieth Street and Broadway since before I was born and would surely be there for decades to come. After I handed Steven a check for $30, he told me Joseph's number. I called later that day.

"That idiot demanded money?" Joseph screamed when I mentioned Steven's broker fee.

We talked for at least an hour. Despite the seriousness of our conversation, I couldn't stop smiling. I knew I had finally found my healer!

Joseph told me one of the reasons so many women get breast cancer. "The lymph."

"Lymph?"

"The lymph carries toxins to the lymph nodes where toxins are filtered out. That's great, but lymph circulates mainly by the physical action of the body, and women's breasts don't move much, confined in those bras you all wear."

I'd never read that. Nobody had ever told me that. That was a good reason not to wear my confounded mastectomy bra.

The PhD in biochemistry told me many new things. "Eat your broccoli . . ." (I'd heard that) ". . . because the indole-3-carbinol . . ." (I'd heard of that) ". . . induces the action of cytochrome P450 and glutathione S-transferase, two major detoxification enzyme systems." I hadn't heard that. I didn't understand a bit of it, but my mind went warm and fuzzy that Joseph did. I was even more impressed that, unlike all the other healers and supposed healers I'd seen, Joseph had cured himself of cancer—of the liver—twenty-one years earlier, using a program of diet and supplements similar to the one he would recommend for me. I couldn't wait to meet him.

I wasn't disappointed. The small two-room apartment in Soho that Joseph shared with his wife was stuffed with shelf after shelf of science and healing books, and stacks of cardboard boxes bulging with bottles of supplements. He was a self-advertisement for his nutritional program, looking twenty years younger than his age of sixty-nine, with a trim physique, thick, wavy gray hair and smooth, pale skin that seemed almost iridescent. He used a sophisticated version of muscle testing to check my health and determine my supplements, all the while sprinkling his talk with Irish, English, Indian, Puerto Rican and Japanese accents, often switching from one to the other in mid-sentence. At first, I found his linguistic virtuosity unsettling—I wasn't looking for Robin Williams—but soon I joined right in. *Pourquoi pas?* I'd found my health plan *and* Robin Williams.

As I watched Joseph write out a detailed chart for my diet and pills, I knew his plan would require just enough of me. I would have to eat intelligently and buy all the pills he recommended, schlep them home and wash them down—sometimes as many as forty a day. But this wouldn't take hours and hours of my time.

Gathering my trench coat and knapsack, I noticed Joseph preparing my bill for my one-and-a-half-hour visit. Oh my God, in all my excitement at finding him, I had forgotten to ask how much he charged—maybe gazillions! "That will be $50, lassie, if ye do not mind," he said with a Scottish lilt.

As I say, Susie stopped appearing on October 3rd. I guess she "integrated" back into me, as Harriet put it, since I was no longer terrified of imminent death. This was healthy, of course, and I know Susie will always be a fundamental part of me. Still, to tell you the truth, I miss her.

Lori went to Joseph once, but said she couldn't trust a man who spoke in accents. Coincidentally, though, her fibroids shrank shortly after she saw him, and they never hurt her again. She was so grateful, she had her own ALTERNATIVE HEALTH INFORMATION BROKER business cards printed up, and in her spare time, started guiding people through the maze of alternative healing herself, at no charge.

Since meeting Joseph, I've never considered looking for another healer. Both he and I continue to be in radiant health. Actually, I think I've always understood that I could follow Joseph's health regimen and still get cancer again or, alternatively, I could do nothing he recommends and never get it again. I think the greatest gift Joseph has been giving me all these years is faith, faith that I will survive, a tangible kind of faith I can swallow every day. Faith has always been important to me.

7 ☙

Of Hands, Purple Herring and Faith

THROUGH THE WINDOW OF THE B&B'S TCHOTCHKE-happy breakfast room, the sky was cloudless, a robin's egg blue. After grabbing our knapsacks—from our separate rooms—Michael and I found ourselves skipping along the sidewalk, laughing in the fresh late March air.

"Thank you so much for coming with me," I said. It felt unspeakably dear to be with Michael the weekend before my mastectomy. Even though we had stopped being lovers several years earlier, the pure-hearted man remained one of my closest friends. We could still talk about almost anything—theater, art, politics, the nut-burying habits of squirrels and now our failed attempts to find new lovers. And hiking was still one of our favorite things to do together.

"Thank you!" he said. I knew he meant this in two ways. He had never been to Kent, Connecticut, before, so he was happy to spend a weekend exploring the woods there. And, very concerned about me, he was eager to do whatever I wanted before my operation.

Having loved the gentle Berkshire Hills for years, I had longed to be consoled by them, reassured by them, before I lost my own AA hillock. The hills seemed like woodland breasts to me now, gushing with glistening streams, covered with calm canopies of branches filling with the sap of life.

Michael and I passed lawns sprouting sprays of crocuses and daffodils, bordered by riots of forsythia. I smiled at my long-legged friend, ahead of me now, as he assumed his hiking demeanor—Nikon strapped around his neck, eyes scanning for compositions, sure-footed and dainty like a deer. I laughed that this was the same man who would be a jumble of arms and legs when we used to occasionally gyrate on the dance floor. The bushes and trees were alive with new sprigs and buds. I felt like a bud about to burst myself. I would be free of cancer in a few days, free to flower for years to come.

But as we started up the side of a road climbing north out of town, my springy mood collapsed. Would I survive the surgery? Would my surgeon get all the cancer? Would life be tolerable as a one-breasted woman? I began to lag behind, slower and slower, head down, kicking piles of roadside leaves—to scatter them, *shatter* them.

Before long, I tripped over what I assumed to be a big rock. This disruption to my angry rhythm incensed me, and I reached beneath the leaves to toss the offense into the woods. But it wasn't a rock. There, on the edge of a quiet country road some ninety miles from my apartment in Manhattan, there, on the weekend before I was to lose my breast, I picked up a piece of concrete statuary, sheered at each end as if broken from a larger work. It was a female nude from the bottom of her neck to the bottom of her ribs, *with her hands crossed over her breasts!* My body seemed to lose its weight, and I was sure it would simply dissolve into the air, if not for the weight of the bust.

It didn't occur to me that finding the bust might have been haphazard chance, that someone just happened to toss it, or it accidentally fell from a truck, and I just happened to stumble upon it. I was sure the incident had been arranged—an incredible outpouring of grace. I felt this with a huge swelling in my heart. Some force of the universe had manifested this fantastic token of sympathy for a centillionth-of-a-speck-of-life me.

My knees wobbled. "Michael!"

He ran back to me.

"Look!"

I put the bust back down on the leaves and we knelt on either side of it. Michael stared at the startling eight-inch form, sweeping his straight black hair off his forehead and wiggling his nose. Such wiggling usually preceded a comment, such as after I'd sing him a new song I'd written for my cabaret act and he'd be trying to think of the nicest possible way to tell me it sucked. But he didn't say a word.

My eyes fixed on the bust's delicate hands. They immediately brought to mind the giant hands I'd often sensed were holding me up over the past weeks, since the rug of my life had been ripped from under me by the diagnosis. Soft, gentle hands they had seemed, light as dawn, safe as a lap. I'd been wondering if they were something I'd been conjuring in my psyche to comfort myself. My fingers trembled as I touched the cold, gray concrete. Maybe the bust is a kind of effusion of those cradling hands, I thought. Maybe I hadn't just imagined them.

Michael volunteered to carry the nine-pound keen in his knapsack as he led us on a loop through the woods—up to a ridge, along it and down again, at one point passing a beaver family's outrageously large house of branches and mud on the side of a pond. I followed along in a daze.

That night my friend Jean from nearby Washington, Connecticut, joined us for pizza. "How lovely," was all she said when we showed her the nude. I think for Jean, who foraged for wild greens for lunch and decorated her apartment with abandoned bird nests, miracles were everyday occurrences.

Michael was a sweetheart to carry the wondrous gift, but he never waxed poetic about it. When we returned to my apartment the next day, he plunked it onto my kitchen table, wiggled his nose and, planting a smile, pronounced, "All yours."

After we kissed good-bye—on the lips but chastely—I sat down to commune with the amazing display of compassion. Immediately, I began to feel waves of caring, of "I'm so sorry" flowing into me, warming every cell to the point where I thought I might burn up. I decided to wrap the bust in something to express my reverence, and also to shield my eyes from its overwhelming presence. All that love, for me? I riffled through a dresser drawer, bypassing many beautiful silk scarves in favor of a simple white cotton pillowcase, scalloped at the open end and printed with rows and rows of pink rosebuds. It had been my mother's. It was sweet yet sturdy, like Ma. Seeing it always filled me with love for her. I folded the case around the bust and placed it in the center of my dresser—love wrapped in love.

There it sat, week after week, nearby but muffled. When I did fold back the pillowcase, very occasionally, it never overflowed with love as it had before. This was more a relief than a disappointment because I didn't feel as desperate to understand it. But I would still cover up the bust quickly. The love it implied continued to unsettle me. I had no framework for it.

Months passed. The shrouded bust gradually faded into the background, along with most of the paraphernalia in my apartment, and I thought less and less of its incredible grace and that of the giant, loving hands it seemed to emanate from.

IN THE SPRING OF 1994, ANOTHER possible outpouring of grace occurred. This time, instead of trying to evade it, I pushed myself to prove the grace was real. I had never attached any significance to the fact that my mastectomy had been performed shortly before Easter, but now, I realized, the second anniversary of my operation was to fall exactly *on* Easter, on the 1,994th anniversary of Jesus' rising from the dead and ascending into heaven.

I called my bro Pete. We'd talked almost weekly since my diagnosis. He'd give me one cancer prevention tip after another from his chiropractor, numerologist, astrologer and douser friends, as well as his shiatsued, rolfed and craniosacraled friends, in Santa Fe.

"This Easter coincidence must be a sign I'll never have to face cancer again!" I rejoiced. My faith that Joseph's regime would keep me safe was obviously not 100 percent.

"Wow, Sue!" Pete said, echoing my enthusiasm.

"And then when I'm ninety-six, I'll be sleeping with the love of my life—we will have been together for years and years—"

"Where, for God's sake, did you meet this love of yours?" Now in his early fifties, Pete was still single, too. He hadn't met anyone new since he had broken up with a woman six months earlier.

"Not a clue," I sighed. "But we'll be sleeping and I'll just peacefully exhale for the last time."

"Not too pleasant for him."

"Jeez, you're right. We'll expire together."

"Much better."

Suddenly I gasped. "Oh, Christ! You think maybe I'm not *eligible* for this Easter boon because I don't consider myself Christian anymore?"

"God can't be discriminatory."

"You'd think. But, for all we know, maybe Christians get boons on Christian holidays, Jews on Jewish ones—like that."

"Sounds a bit intricate," Pete said.

"Outrageous."

I wasn't at all sure the upcoming Easter coincidence was a boon that meant I would live to my nineties, but I was absolutely sure I wanted it to be. After my brother and I hung up, I reviewed my Christian credentials. I was still nostalgic for the love and safety, the ceremony, the sacredness and awe I'd felt at Saint Stephen's Episcopal Church. Every Sunday from when I was seven until thirteen, my mother, wearing a coat over her nightgown, would drive me, and also my sister Nancy and Pete until they were I can't remember how old, to the small, white, steepled building in downtown Armonk, New York, for the children's part of the service and then church school. I loved the Bible stories, which seemed like fluffy clouds of goodness. When I was about ten, I joined the choir. I was ecstatic with the harmonies we altos created with the sopranos, tenors and basses. I couldn't wait to recite the Lord's Prayer each week with the rest of the congregation, always stretching out the word "hal-low-ed" because the sound made my insides feel they were being brushed by the velvet of pussy willows. At some point, wearing a frilly white dress, I was even confirmed as a member of the church.

I adored Saint Stephen's. I'm sure I would have participated much longer, but my parents sent me off to a boarding school. So endedeth my formal Christian life. So beganeth my drifting away.

I continued to feel deep joy each Easter though. The holiday ushered in a fresh beginning, another chance, for Christians and non-Christians alike. Those of us north of the equator were even treated to the reinforcing wonder of warmer weather and new growth. And who could resist the inter-species efforts of rabbits hiding chicken eggs in the grass?

God knows, as an adult I did search for faith. In between flirtations with Hinduism, four varieties of Buddhism, a watered-down Native American spirituality and a boot camp-style humanism, as well as weekends with New Age mystics and spinning with the Sufis, I even tried a Protestant church or two. But the services always made me livid! The music of the hymns was worn out, pat, corny. And the words—"Onward, Christian Soldiers" could have been a theme song for the Crusades. What did the ever-present tag "through Jesus Christ our Lord" *mean*? Did it mean through the example of his life, of his resurrection with its promise of everlasting life, of God's love? Was Jesus forever begging God to do our bidding? I simply couldn't buy that Jesus was a sacrificial lamb, and that all our supposedly hellish sins and thoroughly sinful natures were forgiven by his death, as if his death were on one side of a scale balancing out some two thousand years of our otherwise unforgivable sins. I couldn't buy that Jesus was the *only* child of God either. The rest of us were liverwurst?

Despite all this bad blood between Christianity and me, when the possibly grace-filled Easter of 1994 arrived, I did want to party. Busy as a bunny, I crisscrossed Manhattan to give Celestina, Michael and two other friends a Godiva chocolate egg. "Before you eat it," I told each of them, "think of something you really, really want." Then I hurried home. Sitting at my kitchen table with a mug of chamomile tea, I made my own wish—that the day was the omen I'd hoped for—and ever so slowly ate my own chocolate egg, letting each small bite melt completely in my mouth. The egg, the size a chicken would lay, was hollow inside as if it had been waiting to be filled with intent.

But how could I be sure my wish would come true? I opened a spiral notebook, picked up a pen and went straight to the source:

ME. I know it's a busy day for you, but *please* tell me, does this Easter coincidence mean that, even though I'm not exactly Christian at the moment, I'll never get cancer again, I won't die of it?

GOD. Susan, Susan, Susan. You could die crossing the street, swallowing a chicken bone, in an airplane crash, a train crash. You could drown, fall down some stairs. . . .

(ME *retreated to her bed.*)

GOD. You could be struck by lightning even here, you know, or be shot—

ME. Excuse me, am I safe from cancer?

GOD. Not necessarily. Maybe. It depends on so many forces, currents, actualizations.

ME. But you planted my anniversary on Easter!

GOD. A bit self-centered, aren't we? Celebrations occur every day of the year for one thing or another somewhere. January one—

ME. But we're talking about Easter, God, resurrection. It's got to mean something.

GOD. Grace happens all the time, dear. And, of course, the minute you sincerely intend something, the universe tends to respond and help you.

ME. You mean swallowing all my supplements has something to do with my anniversary landing on Easter—

GOD. I didn't say that.

ME. Even though I'm not exactly Christian?

GOD. Grace isn't discriminatory.

ME. That's what my brother said.

GOD. You really want to stay alive, don't you?

ME. I haven't experienced nearly enough love and joy yet, nearly enough giving, success.

GOD. I agree with you.

ME. You do?

GOD. You have the potential for much more.

ME. Yes? So you'll let me live to realize it all, right?

GOD. I didn't say that. Everything depends on so many forces, currents, actualizations.

ME. Back to that.

GOD didn't reveal much. Funny how She/He/It spoke in a vernacular so similar to my own.

But I didn't give up on the Easter coincidence. Not me. One day it popped into my brain that I might find confirmation in the Bible that the coincidence meant my redemption. I perused the religion section of the Barnes and Noble on Broadway, looking for a version of the Bible not hopelessly hip, but fresher than the gold-edged King James my Psalms-quoting uncle had sent me years earlier.

It seemed pointless to look further when I came across *The Five Gospels*. According to this slim paperback, Jesus didn't say 82 percent of the words ascribed to him in the Gospels! Now, I didn't consciously rely on Jesus' supposed words, but that he'd said them had been part of the cultural bedrock of much of the Western world, of my world in an unexamined way. The bedrock had just collapsed.

I collapsed into one of the cushy bookstore chairs. Sheila must know about this, I thought. I'd met with the young Episcopalian minister, a friend of a friend, the week before to get her professional opinion on my Easter coincidence. She had been curt and businesslike—and maddeningly noncommittal—until she leaned back against her upright wooden chair and started crying. "God must love us so much to send his Son to earth to teach the truth. Jesus must love us so much to have died for us," she managed between sobs. I sat in a matching upright chair on the other side of her large, gray metal desk, fighting back tears at the depth of her faith—a depth of spiritual connection or at least aliveness I envied.

I rubbed my hand with and against the tan corduroy nap of the bookstore chair. Sheila was a recent graduate of Yale Divinity School. She was employed by a high-end church on the Upper East Side. She must know about the 82 percent. She must know she is responding to mostly myth. Sheila seemed to confirm something I remembered the famous scholar Joseph Campbell saying, that myths, "the music of the spheres" as he called them, survive because they respond to human longings, the soul's longings.

Could the mythical Bible possibly speak to my longing too? I grabbed a King James off the Barnes and Noble Bible shelf, curled up in the comfy chair and poured through the New Testament. Some of the archaic language was beautiful. But none of it even hinted at any boon on Easter—except for Jesus rising from his death. I guess that was enough of a boon for one day. But a sentence I saw in the Gospel of Luke (and Luke only— the Gospels, I was discovering, were shockingly inconsistent) began to swim in my head. It was ascribed to Jesus right before he died on the Cross, although he didn't really say it according to *The Five Gospels*—oh, well. "Father, into thy hands I commit my spirit," Luke's Jesus said. "Into thy hands I commit. ..." Luke's Jesus must have been filled with God's love for him. "Into thy hands. . . . " I remembered the giant, caring hands I'd felt carrying me after I was diagnosed and the compassionate concrete hands that had appeared at my feet. The grace of these hands had filled my heart effortlessly.

In contrast, the Easter coincidence had led me to incessant pondering. Enough already! I tossed the Bible to the floor. The coincidence had been just haphazard chance, as GOD had hinted, a paschal purple herring.

But the hands—they couldn't be haphazard. I rushed home to look at the bust. I hadn't unwrapped it in months.

The worry line between my eyebrows squeezed tight as I hesitantly pulled back Ma's rosebud pillowcase. Would the weighty form still unglue me with awe? No. Now the sight of it actually relaxed me. Its slender hands seemed to caress the breasts as though this were the most natural activity in the world, as though caressing were at the heart of everything. I felt the love of the hands as a fact as solid as concrete, and as soft as pussy willows.

I called Jean the next day.

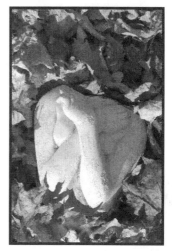

"Maybe it's time for you to let the bust go, let someone else find it," she suggested.

I've thought about doing this. I have. But every time I look at the concrete hands, I feel that love. I don't know how long I will live, but I know I am loved. And who am I? A centillionth of a speck of life. Not even.

8 ৵

A Rash of Procedures

CONTINUING TO POP JOSEPH'S REGIMEN OF PILLS, I thought of myself as brimming with health in the fall of 1994. But as the brilliance of the leaves faded, on the morning of Wednesday, November 2nd, according to my appointment book, I noticed a peculiar area of brilliance on me: five blood-red dots on my ribs. At nine a.m. sharp I dialed my health guru.

"Always get symptoms checked out by the medical establishment," Joseph advised.

Thus began a month of more diagnostic procedures than I'd ever had in my life.

As soon as Joseph and I hung up, I called my dermatologist.

"The dots are probably nothing," she said, "but with your cancer history, I should see them."

"SKIN CANCER," my mind screamed.

After we hung up, it occurred to me that as a cancer survivor, I should be vigilant about other bodily oddities I was ignoring. My period, for example, was starting every two weeks. I called my gynecologist.

"It's probably only beginning menopause," Dr. Collins said. I'd turned fifty in September. "But I want to see you, just to be sure."

"UTERINE CANCER!"

I'd also had abdominal pain for weeks and had been burping so much I thought I might morph into a frog. Since I was clerking for a gastroenterologist, I asked him for some free advice.

"With your history, we should check it out. I'll give you a colonoscopy," Dr. Slattery decided.

"COLON CANCER!"

While I had my boss's attention—a rare occurrence—I also asked him about some stiffness I'd been having in my fingers and knees. He referred me to a rheumatologist buddy of his.

I STARED AT MYSELF IN MY bathroom mirror that night. Is this what a "professional" patient looks like?

MY GYN INSERTED AN INSTRUMENT INTO my somewhat desiccated and hence *sensitive* vagina to take a biopsy of my uterus and, with the instrument still in my vagina, announced, "Huh, a polyp."

"VAGINAL CANCER!"

Dr. Collins cut out the polyp and then, my insides writhing with cramps, resumed her pursuit, through my miniscule cervix, to my shrunken uterus where she—pow!—snagged a piece of it. She sent the polyp and the uterine specimen off to a lab.

As I lay recovering on the exam table, feet still in stirrups, I asked Dr. Collins if she thought I should get my left ovary checked out. No doubt also shrunken by now, it was especially dear to me since when I was sixteen my right ovary was removed due to a cyst.

"Absolutely," she said immediately. "We'll get a sonogram."

The next day, my dermatologist assured me that all my red dots were just part of the aging process. Now that was a new one, but, hey, I *was* aging. That was good. But as she was looking me over, she noticed an irregularly shaped freckle on the back of my right leg.

"SKIN CANCER!"

She cut it off and sent it to a lab. "Just to be sure," she said lightly. "It's probably nothing."

She began to rub one of her fingers back and forth over my left shoulder.

"What?" I asked.

"It's probably nothing, but you should have it removed."

"Okay." She kept rubbing. Why wasn't she fetching her knife? "Let's do it," I urged.

"Not me. You need a surgeon. I handle things on the skin, not under it."

Where would specialization end?

Under the skin.

"BONE CANCER!"

I scheduled the surgery with a friend of my boss's.

Meanwhile I had the sonogram of my left ovary, a relatively benign procedure except that I had to drink a quart of water beforehand, and when the technician pressed her probe down on my abdomen—wherein is located my bladder—I almost let loose. The following day my GYN called to tell me my ovary had a "calcification."

To someone whose breast cancer had been detected by "micro-calcifications" on a mammogram, this sounded very, very bad.

"OVARIAN CANCER!"

Dr. Collins was cautiously optimistic. "It's probably nothing, but let's get an MRI just to be sure."

"An MRI!" I knew Magnetic Resonance Imaging machines were like mummy cases. "I feel claustrophobic walking through an underpass in Central Park!"

"No problem," she said. "We'll find you an open MRI. They give you plenty of room."

I was ambivalent the following day as my boss performed my colonoscopy. Drugged enough not to be anxious, I lay on my right side and watched the scope's progress on a screen. There was my colon, a sudden video star in vivid color. But the scope was giving me abdominal cramps, and my rear end, until this moment always covered at the office in one demure way or another, was in my boss's face. "You have a small polyp in your ascending colon," Dr. Slattery said.

"COLON CANCER!"

"I'm sure it's nothing," he continued. He cut it out and directed his nurse to send it to a lab. "You also have hemorrhoids."

Yuk.

LYING HAZY-HEADED IN THE RECOVERY room, I sensed that the white blanket was separating my mind from the rest of my body, as if my body were an independent entity. It has a will of its own, I thought. What will it come up with next? Maybe I'm overreacting, I countered. Maybe all my physical oddities are within the normal range of variability for a body still walking and talking after five decades. Am I being a neurotic hypochondriac milking my medical insurance? But cancer survivors have to be wary. I remembered a survivor who told me that when she'd found a tiny bump on her index finger, she had it checked by five different specialists. And it was my doctors who recommended all the procedures, hopefully out of concern for me. Of course, they also must have been worried about malpractice suits, as well as delighted to refer patients to their buddies in the spirit of reciprocity.

THREE DAYS LATER, I CALLED MY GYN for lab results on the uterine biopsy and the vaginal polyp. Both negative.

"YES!"

I called my dermatologist about the biopsy of the freckle she'd removed from my leg. Negative.

"YES!"

Feeling almost cocky, I trotted over to Park Avenue late that afternoon for the MRI.

"Don't worry," the MRI technician said glibly as my eyes popped at the off-white seven-foot cube in the basement of the radiology office. In the middle of the cube was a slit, no more than six feet wide and one and a half feet high, *no more*, from which protruded a stretcher on wheels. The buff young man fluffed the pillow at the end of the stretcher like a doting Delta steward. "What kind of music would you like?" Dixieland jazz was already playing.

I was still focused on the stretcher. "How far in will my head be?"

"A few inches." He gestured for me to lie down and then strapped a silver belt over my abdomen.

I would definitely need a distraction. But the Dixieland made me want to get up and boogie. "Do you have any classical music?"

"Sure. People love the Mozart." The steward was all smiles as he wheeled me in.

There couldn't have been more than *three inches* from the top of me to the top of the space, and the crown of my head was about *two feet* inside the machine. Liar! I twisted my head to glare at him, but he was walking briskly toward the door. A knot formed in my stomach. I broke into a sweat. "I don't think I can do this," I whimpered.

"You'll be fine. I'll be right behind the wall. Just follow my instructions."

The door closed.

For a split second, the room seemed vacuumed of sound, and my mind flashed back to the completely empty house I once performed before, at midnight, at a one-act festival in a theater near Bloomingdale's. But then my ears tuned to the rambunctious jazz again. My toes started wiggling to it. When was he going to change the music! My neck ached from craning toward the door, so I turned my head around to rest it squarely on the pillow. Oh my God, the tiny clearance above me had shrunk. The machine was going to *smoosh* me into a crêpe any second!

"Don't move, Miss Cummings."

I froze my toes and closed my eyes. God! God! (Why didn't I direct my pleading to the huge, compassionate hands? I guess I thought I needed more than hands.) God! God, be with me! God, be with me! God? God? I know I'm going to be alright. This is a good thing. They'll find out if my ovary is okay.

The gigantic machine came alive above me. "Dat, dat, dat, dat, dat, dat, dat, dat," it said, like rapidly firing bullets. "Dat, dat, dat, dat, dat, dat, dat, dat."

"Breathe in, Miss Cummings. Hold it. Breathe out. Breathe in. Hold it. Breathe out. . . . "

That incessant, let's-have-a-party jazz! I told him I wanted the Mozart! Keep calm. Keep calm. God? God!

"Dat, dat, dat, dat, dat, dat, dat, dat."

God? God! Lily Tomlin. Lily Tomlin? Lily Tomlin! Lily Tomlin in a drawer. Yes! She's tiny, like I saw her years ago on TV, sitting in a huge stuffed chair, only now she's lying in a great big drawer. Yes! *I* am tiny Lily Tomlin in the king-size drawer.

I am tiny Lily Tomlin in the drawer. Don't let my mind wander, not for a second. I am getting a good night's sleep in the drawer. I am teeny Lily Tomlin in the enormous drawer. I am Lily Tomlin sleeping happily on a soft down comforter in the gargantuan drawer. I am Lily Tomlin dreaming sweet dreams in the city block of a drawer. I am Lily Tom. . . . "

"It's all over, Miss Cummings," the technician said. I hadn't heard him come into the room. He released the stretcher, and I let out bellows-like pants as if I'd just finished the New York City marathon.

Two afternoons later, I lay on my right side on an operating room table, fully awake, as the surgeon, assisted by his nurse, cut out the growth on my shoulder and sent it for analysis. I heard the following:

"Did you have fun at Mark's party?" Dr. Posusta asked her.

"Karl was there," she responded.

"Yes?"

"With his new girlfriend."

"He can be so tactless."

"So I accidentally spilled my entire glass of red wine all over his suit."

"You're terrible."

I didn't want to interrupt to ask how my procedure was going.

AS SOON AS DR. POSUSTA SEWED me up, I took the subway to Penn Station. I would spend Thanksgiving in Princeton with Marge, my father's second wife, now his widow. Daddy had died in early October of a rare lung disease. Marge and I had been on either side of his bed when he tossed and turned for the last time.

It was a comfort to be with Marge, for us to mourn together. We shared stories about Daddy, read magazines, watched

Big Bird and Kermit the Frog float down Broadway on TV. I usually found these overblown characters charmless, ludicrous, proof that bigger is frequently not better. But this Thanksgiving they seemed to be audacious, seemed in a way to be commemorating Daddy, a bigger than life character himself—six foot five, a commanding presence in any room.

Before the turkey breast with gravy, mashed potatoes and salad, Marge and I declared, as was Marge and Daddy's custom, "Blessings on the meal." Marge added, "God, bless Bart."

I fought back the tears. I'd had such a conflicted relationship with the man. He hadn't been the father I'd wanted, and I hadn't been the daughter he'd wanted. But I would always hold in my heart the simple part of him that enjoyed a family outing of fishing and picnicking along the banks of the Moose River in the Adirondacks.

Over pumpkin pie, I gave silent thanks that my test results were all negative so far. I wish I could say that I reevaluated my medical situation during my hiatus from the city, that mourning my father's death in the condo where he had died slowed me down, mellowed me, cured me of scurrying from specialist to specialist. Such scurrying hadn't cured my father. But, in fact, I think being with Marge and breathing in Daddy's lingering vapors made me even more anxious to keep my own death at bay.

MY COLON POLYP RESULTS WERE DELIVERED to Dr. Slattery's office the following Monday. Negative.

"THANK GOD!"

"I think we should have a urologist check out your abdominal pain," Dr. Slattery said. He sent me that very morning to a buddy of his across the street.

With my history, Dr. Chinn said, just to be sure, he'd like to examine my bladder by performing a "cystoscopy."

"BLADDER CANCER!"

"You could have it done in a hospital with anesthesia," he explained, "but anesthesia is really unnecessary. It would be much faster and simpler to do it right here in my office."

"Okay." What did I know?

Four days later Dr. Posusta called me at Dr. Slattery's with the lab results of the shoulder growth. Negative.

"THANK GOD!"

After we hung up, I called my GYN.

"The MRI didn't show anything," Dr. Collins said.

I waited for her to continue her sentence with something like "so you can relax."

"That's good, right?" I asked.

"Well, MRIs are usually good at picking up ovaries, but unfortunately that open MRI was not. I need to send you for a CAT scan."

I articulated very slowly through clenched teeth, "You mean I didn't need to go through that MRI?"

"I suppose you could look at it that way."

Still steaming after work, I stormed across town to see the rheumatologist. He asked a few questions, put me through some range-of-motion tests and said, "Well, with your history, I recommend a bone scan, just to be sure."

"BONE CANCER!"

If one more person said, "Just to be sure"!

At the radiologist's office for the bone scan the next day, a nurse asked me to sign a consent form before I drank a large cup of thick milkshake-like glop. According to the form, the glop was laced with technetium-99, which would apparently circulate through my blood to all my bones.

"Is technetium-99 related to strontium-90?" I asked her.

"It's radioactive, if that's what you mean. But, not to worry—it decays quickly."

"Uh-huh. But will it decay me quickly?"

She smiled quickly and pointed to the signature line.

I read wholesome *Reader's Digest* stories in the reception area for three hours, the prescribed time for the technetium-99 to charge all my bones, and then a monotonic technician, with the cordiality a secretary would grant a new eraser, led me into a room and directed me to lie down on a cold, gray metal table. I noticed the big black block suspended from the ceiling at the end of the table, but didn't think much about it.

"Find a comfortable position and don't move."

"Okay."

The big black block began to move down from the ceiling to, I was sure, an eighth of an inch above my feet. Then the big black block began to advance up over the rest of my body, slowly, relentlessly, like a two-ton snail.

A tsunami of claustrophobia flooded me again. The monster snail was going to squish me into two-dimensionality. My eyes were glued to the block. Now it was approaching my knees. "I can't do this!" I yelled.

"I'll be here with you," the technician said in her robot-speak.

Lucky me.

The block continued toward my thighs. I considered slipping off the table, but my body was frozen. Even my sweat glands were frozen. I stopped breathing. "Let me out!" I screamed.

The technician immediately called out, "Izzy," and I heard someone enter so fast she must have been on call on the other side of the door. Izzy dragged a chair over to me, sat and slid one of her hands over mine on the table. I grabbed onto her short fingers and held tight. "Not to worry, I'm right here," she said in a warm, refreshingly modulated Puerto Rican accent. My eyes darted toward her—barely past her teens, the whites of her large, dark eyes highlighted by liner, her hair a mass of black curls, a broad smile on her fuchsia-painted lips. I closed my eyes, focused on Izzy's soft, cool hand, and immediately calmed down. Another hand.

Afterwards, I hugged Izzy four times.

The results, which a radiologist was kind enough to tell me half an hour later: "Normal—a little arthritis and some benign bone islands." The islands were areas of compact bone, he explained.

"THANK GOD!"

Compact bone sounded healthy.

On my way to work a few days later, I had the CAT scan for my shy ovary—an unremarkable event, really, except for the exposure to an untold number of X-rays.

During lunch, I dashed across the street to have Dr. Chinn perform his cystoscopy. When he began to wiggle some tubing up my extremely narrow urethra to my bladder, without the "unnecessary" anesthesia, my body immediately began to sweat all over the way it does when I'm about to faint, which I am wont to do when experiencing *extreme pain*. Without thinking about it, I started humming. The gentle vibrations from the sound were amazingly soothing. I actually became tranquil. I was so busy humming, I didn't hear Dr. Chinn at first.

"Miss Cummings, Miss Cummings, you can stop humming now."

"Oh."

"Everything looks good."

"THANK GOD!"

My GYN called the next morning with the results of the CAT scan of my ovary. "Everything's fine. The calcifications are benign."

"YES!"

UPON WAKING ONE MORNING IN MID-DECEMBER, I rolled from my usual sleeping position on my right side onto my back, clasped my hands over my ribs and smiled up at the rosy pink ceiling. Not only had my abdominal pain, the burping and the stiffness in my joints all disappeared without any intervention, but neither I nor anyone else had discovered a new physical symptom in more than a week!

What, pray tell, had all the symptoms and procedures meant? Since every result came out negative, I thought, all the procedures had been in a sense *unnecessary*. I definitely wished I'd skipped the ones I could use some day to prepare for roles in which I am tortured. The toxic ones might subtract days from my life. But, I had to admit, the procedures had strengthened my faith in Joseph's regimen and also in comforting hands. Additionally, I now had greater appreciation for activities usually considered fairly useless. Pretending to be tiny and humming like a motor can turn out to be very handy. You never know.

The month had been an emotional elevator ride, down and up, down and up, between purgatory and salvation. With every negative test result, I felt the surge of being granted a new chance at life. It was as though my body had been taken apart, organ by organ, and put back together much stronger, healthier and happier. I felt radiant. Never mind that some of that radiance might be radioactive.

Springing out of bed, I vowed never again to subject my body to those scalpels, probes, poisons and monolithic blocks. I had my own procedures. I unbottled the twenty-two supplements Joseph recommended I take with breakfast and filled a glass of water from my Shaklee triple filter to wash them down. I fixed my usual bowl of organic oatmeal and plain organic yogurt, sweetened with vegetable glycerine. But this morning I fortified my porridge with a hearty spoonful each of organic pumpkin seeds, organic walnuts, organic raisins, organic flaxseeds, organic flaxseed oil and chlorella flakes, as well as a sliced-up organic Granny Smith apple and two dropperfuls of concentrated decaffeinated green tea. Just to be sure.

9 ⪫

Who Needs Affirmations?

I WAS LAZING BENEATH MY COZY ROSY PINK POLYESTER comforter one cold morning later that December, gazing through half-opened eyes at the rosy pink walls and ceiling of my bedroom. I'd been enjoying this placidity, not unlike a hibernating bear, for some time, with nary a thought—not even one cursing my landlord for being a stingy SOB with the heating oil, certainly not one reeking of self-improvement.

Rrrrring! Rrrrring!

I checked the time on my alarm clock and jolted out of bed. Who calls anyone in New York at eight on a Sunday? Something must be terribly wrong. Donning my down robe, I clopped in my sheepskin slippers to the phone in the kitchen.

"Hello?"

"Susan!"

It was Diana. She and I had become fast friends after we'd met at a breast cancer survivor workshop in New York about a year earlier. "What's the matter?"

"Listen to this! 'Breasts represent mothering and nurturing.' And here's an affirmation for them: 'I take in and give out nourishment in perfect balance.'"

Despite the kitchen's whiteness, I began to see red as I suspected where Diana was headed. "That's odd," I said. "I thought breasts represent hatred and fear."

She ignored me. "When you combine that with what this book says are some of the probable causes of cancer—'Deep hurt. Long-lasting resentment.'—no wonder we got breast cancer, huh? I feel like she's talking to us!"

"Diana! I'm not listening to some kook tell us why we got cancer! How the hell would she know?" I slammed my hand down on the kitchen table. "Sorry. Guess I got out of the wrong side of the bed. Of course, since my bed's against the wall, I can only get out the one side."

Diana giggled.

"Listen, can I call you when I get out again, say at eleven?"

"She wrote a whole book, Susan."

"Just because it's written, doesn't make it true, hon. Lots of people aren't nurturing and hold resentments, but they don't get cancer."

"So why do *you* think you got it?"

"I don't know. But I don't want to feel guilty about it, like I did something wrong." Pulling my robe around me tighter, I sat down at my kitchen table. "Diana, please. Don't blame yourself for your recurrence." Diana had had a bout with cancer in her left breast nine years earlier. It had been treated by a lumpectomy, radiation and chemotherapy, but now the cancer was back, not only in her breast but also her left cheekbone, sternum, lower back and one lung.

"I don't know if blame is exactly the right word."

"Diana, don't go there, okay? What good does it do? And it's so humiliating—like everyone's thinking, 'They must be so unevolved. That's why they got cancer.'"

"But what about your father?"

"What about him?"

"You have a lot of resentment toward him, don't you?"

She was right. I still did. It amazed me. He had died over two months earlier. I loved him, I admired him, but I was still angry at his relentless criticism of me. His ultimate put-down kept looping in my mind. "I don't even tell new friends I have a second daughter," he told me once when I was visiting in Princeton. My resentment felt very heavy, dark, ugly.

But while I knew psychological states could affect the physical body—I sometimes got a cold when I was stressed out—the idea that my resentment could cause cancer seemed ludicrous. I didn't put it quite this way to Diana. "Please, it's not like I'm gonna let go of my resentment any time soon."

"Maybe you can. Listen to her affirmations for cancer:

I lovingly forgive and release all of the past.
I choose to fill my world with joy.
I love and approve of myself.

Aren't they wonderful? She says to write them down or say them out loud into a mirror."

I took a deep breath and exhaled slowly. I'd tried affirmations. Once I wrote "I am a successful actress" and "I am in a wonderful relationship with a man" twenty-five times a day for three weeks. Sometimes I'd get quite elaborate, jotting down negative thoughts that had occurred to me as I was doing the affirming and then countering these negatives with additional affirmations. The only changes I created were more paper waste, more profits for paper and pen companies and hand cramps.

Maybe writing affirmations didn't work for me because I was skeptical of simple statements. I'd grown up hearing my

father discuss advertising slogans for products that were practically identical to other products—"Look, Ma, no cavities!"
I myself, both as a writer and an actress, had manipulated
words for years to suit my own purposes. In any case, I found
the rote repetition of untruths a silly waste of time. "If they
help you, dear, I'm glad, I really, really am," I told my friend
who so needed and deserved hope.

"It's Louise Hay, Susan. She's a cancer survivor."

"There are a number of us. Listen, sweetie, would you
mind if I called you later?"

After we hung up, I shuffled back to bed and tried to re-
sume my communion with rosy pink, but guilt took over. I
was such a lousy friend. So what if I didn't believe in affirmations? I should have been more supportive of Diana. I was
in a very different situation than she. I had had a mastectomy
for stage zero breast cancer and so far hadn't had to deal with
more disease. It was totally understandable that she would
try affirmations. She wanted to do everything possible for
herself—outside of conventional treatment. She refused to
go the slash-burn-poison route this time. God, I hoped she'd
make it. She could, she could. I'd read of people surviving
metastases.

About three weeks later, Diana and I, both loverless, decided to celebrate Valentine's Day together. She greeted me at the
door of her funky fourth-floor walk-up on East Eighty-fifth
Street in her dungaree skirt and bright red woolen turtleneck.
I was shocked, as usual, at how fresh she looked at forty-two,
with her smooth skin and shiny chestnut hair and a smile that
seemed to extend halfway around her head. Despite the pain
I knew she was experiencing in her cheek, sternum and back,
her face looked especially light and calm that afternoon, as if
she'd just come from an hour of sailing. At the same time, her
slender five-foot-seven frame appeared to claim more space

than usual.

We sat at her kitchen table and devoured two pieces each of the organic carob cake with carob icing she'd made.

"This is delicious!" I said. "I think I almost prefer carob to chocolate now."

"I wouldn't go that far."

I gave her a gift certificate to Joseph Fischl, an art supply store on Third Avenue, since I knew she wanted to get back into painting. She'd done very little since she'd majored in art at Hunter College.

Tearing away the shiny red wrapping paper, I gasped when I saw what she gave me: *You Can Heal Your Life* by Louise Hay. Most of the cover was filled with a bright rainbow shaped into a heart. "Diana, you shouldn't have!"

We both laughed.

"I know you think it's a shitty present, but I just had to get it for you." She reached across the table and placed one of her hands over mine. "Please don't let what happened to me happen to you, Susan. I'm convinced cancer doesn't just happen." She proceeded to chide herself for not heeding her wake-up call nine years ago, reiterating how she should have found time to paint, should have quit the word processing job she hated, should have divorced her rage-aholic ex-husband years earlier. What she regretted most was not getting her schizophrenic daughter, Sandy, now sixteen, into a group home much sooner. She used to get so depressed from all this, she said, that she'd polish off a pound cake at least once a week.

"Oh, Diana, I really don't think. . . . " I didn't want her to berate herself, but I became speechless when it hit me that *my* life wasn't exactly a bundle of joy at the moment, was it? Supposedly an actress, I hadn't auditioned since I was diagnosed. Would I live out the rest of my days as a part-time clerk for a gastroenterologist? Would I always live in my 300-square-foot walk-up apartment, just me, my spider plant and the barks from the poor pooches in the Bark Avenue Boutique on the first floor?

"I promise I won't nag you about Louise any more," Diana said. "It's just that I'm finding her book so helpful." She told me she was now repeating affirmations in the mirror every day and doing mental exercises Ms. Hay recommended to forgive her ex-husband. And she'd started working with Dale, a non-traditional healer she'd found in Westchester who was "brilliant" and also "a hunk."

So, all this explained her peace and confidence. My eyes welled with tears at her positive mindset. "Wow, that's all wonderful, hon!"

Filled with admiration and affection for Diana, as soon as I returned home, I tried reading *You Can Heal Your Life*. I made it to page five.

"We create every so-called 'illness' in our body."

"Releasing resentment will dissolve even cancer."

Bull___! I hurled the book across the living room. But then, touched by it coming from Diana, I squeezed it into the top shelf of one of my bookcases.

For various reasons, Diana and I didn't talk for several weeks, and when I did call, I got her mother, who was visiting from Florida to help out. She said that she'd be going back home in a few days because, even though Diana was getting weaker, she'd moved in with Dale. Weaker? Dale? I had to see her.

"Welcome to Shangri-la North!" Diana said at the door of Dale's small white cape in Rye, a short train ride north of the city. She'd lived in Manhattan since her twenties, so I guess a house on a quiet suburban cul-de-sac seemed idyllic, especially with three flowering maples in the front yard. Her beige cotton shirtwaist fit her like a muumuu and she felt practically fleshless when I hugged her, but she seemed filled with delight, like a Persian cat who could perceive only pleasure.

We settled on the lumpy gray couch in the living room. Dale came in, a handsome fellow about Diana's age and height. Preppily dressed in creased khakis and a crisp, light-blue oxford shirt, he looked too conformist to be the chemist who, Diana had told me, had been treating cancer patients illegally for six years. He stood next to her at the end of the couch and ran his fingers slowly through her hair. His own curly dark hair would frequently flop over his left eye and he would flip it back with a quick toss of his head. The well-worn furnishings in the room, handed down from his mother, Dale explained, were interspersed with treatment machines that resembled serious Pilates apparatuses fitted with chemistry lab glassware. Dale said he had imported them from Germany.

"You hear that?" Diana asked, looking toward the window at the far end of the room. We all smiled at the swell of cheery chirps coming from Dale's backyard, probably from a flock of early spring arrivals. Diana sighed contentedly. "Living here and being in love—really for the first time and with such a gifted healer—I can't help but get better, don't you think?" She beamed up at Dale.

"Absolutely," Dale said.

"Yes!" I said, shaking my arm in a hurrah, my heart begging that it would be so.

Diana only alluded to Louise Hay once during my weekly visits. "I don't need to say affirmations anymore," she said lightly one afternoon, propped up with pillows in bed. She looked paler than I'd ever seen her. "My most important ones have come true."

What about "I am healed from cancer!" I wanted to protest from the bedside chair. Why don't you affirm that? Are you accepting, even embracing, death? But Diana's smile looked so serene, I said nothing and smiled back.

A few weeks went by. Diana got weaker and weaker.

Dale called one morning in early May to tell me she had died in her sleep. It wasn't that I hadn't expected it. But she was in midlife, for God's sake, and in love. I felt I'd lost a sister.

You liar, Louise Hay! Releasing resentments can't dissolve cancer. Diana said her affirmations night and day until shortly before she died. She didn't have an ounce of resentment left in her.

So much for affirmations.

IN JUNE, MY THERAPIST HARRIET MOVED to Santa Fe, and I began seeing a "life coach," aka unlicensed therapist, whom I'd met at a women's support group. After I told Alice a little about myself at my first session, she revealed that she too had had breast cancer. What a coincidence, I thought. Though I was sorry that she had had to face the disease, I looked forward to deep empathy between us. Then she launched into elaborate praise of Louise Hay! Diana must be laughing, I thought. Alice said she consulted *You Can Heal Your Life* daily and thought Ms. Hay was right on about why she got the disease.

"I will not discuss why I got breast cancer," I almost shouted. "I want to work on my crap, but I will not entertain the possibility that my crap caused my cancer. Period."

When I had an earache in July, Alice pulled *You Can Heal Your Life* from the bookshelf beside her chair.

"I don't want to hear it."

She put the book back and started laughing.

"What?"

"I bet that's what earaches represent: not wanting to hear."

"Everyone who gets an earache doesn't want to hear?"

"Well. . . . "

Despite her pig-headedness about Louise Hay, I was very grateful to have found Alice. She was intuitive as well as bright, always caring, and she clarified aspects of my life that had been mush to me for years. She certainly *talked* her talk, constantly repeating affirmations to improve her relationships with herself, her family and her God, and to become a better and richer life coach. Affirmations seemed to be working for her. Still, even as I moaned that I couldn't get myself back to auditioning and hadn't had a date since before I was diagnosed, I pooh-poohed them. One day I actually screamed, "Pa-leeease! No more Louise!" To no avail. Alice continued to plug them.

Meanwhile, my brother Pete, who had managed his manic-depression fairly successfully with lithium for years, was in a deep depression. By September, he'd been battling it for seven months. He was doing everything he could to recover—seeing a therapist, trying different prescription drugs his doctor recommended, praying, meditating twice a day, hosting a weekly men's support group. But most of the time he lay on his couch reading mysteries. As I heard his slow, flat voice one day in September, I felt desperate to help.

They popped into my head. They couldn't hurt him. At least they'd give him something else to do. "Have you heard of affirmations?"

"Yeah, sure. I affirm I'm fucking sick of being depressed!"

"Listen, I know it sounds stupid but—I don't know—this Louise Hay says if you say positive statements of things you want in your life, this will help you create them. 'I am happy, thriving and energetic.' Like that."

"I don't know, Sue...."

I was determined to motivate him. "Hey," I said, flabbergasted, "we'll both do it—think up four positive affirmations and say them, looking at ourselves in the mirror—that's supposed to be very important—every day for a week."

"You'll do it too?"

What had I gotten myself into? "Yes."

I called Pete a week later. He wasn't over his depression, but he said he enjoyed saying his affirmations and planned to continue. It might have been my imagination, but I thought there was more modulation in his voice.

I couldn't believe it, but I enjoyed saying my affirmations too, looking at myself right in the eyeballs. I'd come up with five:

> I love and accept myself exactly as I am.
> I am healthy physically, psychologically and
>   spiritually.
> I am a capable, worthwhile and successful artist.
> I give and receive love abundantly.
> I am in a life-long, intimate relationship with
>   a man, that is happy, healthy, loving, sexy and
>   stimulating.

I'd put a lot of thought into the details of that last one—an utter impossibility.

Saying my Pollyanna sentences made me feel embarrassed at first, like a brainwashed convert to a positive thinking cult. I also felt I was violating something, as though I were a director giving the actress—also me—totally new lines to a play that had been set for years. Who did I think I was? God? Repeating the statements to my reflection in the mirror was much more powerful than writing them down. All of me seemed to be talking to all of me. Sometimes my eyes would overflow with tears from longing, and also from momentarily believing my affirmations were true.

My life didn't change dramatically at first. But after less than a month of affirming, my resentment of my father felt more like a memory. He had done the best he could. New ways of being in the world began to seem vaguely possible. I felt more capable and worthy, more optimistic and also simply content.

Alice was thrilled that I was finally affirming. Oh, how I wished I could tell Diana. Maybe she knows.

10 ✍

Pennies from Heaven

"ARE YOU WALKING THIS SUNDAY?" CELESTINA ASKED. My friend was looking across the subway aisle at a poster in pink and purple lettering.

I rolled my eyes in disgust. The American Cancer Society was promoting its October 1995 "Making Strides Against Breast Cancer Walk." "Absolutely not," I barked.

Sprawled in our seats, Celestina and I had been tapping our feet, still grooving to the smooth sounds of the Lou Donaldson Quartet we'd just heard at the Vanguard. We'd treated ourselves to the set at this cellar shrine to jazz in the Village in order to forget for an hour or so the state of our affairs—the lack thereof. Celestina had just had a disastrous date with a man she'd have to kiss for weeks in an off-Broadway play. He had turned out to be an unstoppable monologist offstage. My daily affirming that I had found the love of my life had so far only resulted in a few hot-to-trot fantasies.

As it turned out, the quartet's velvety instrumentals, especially its second to last number, embraced Celestina's and my respective sadnesses and gently modulated them into dreamy hope. "Every time it rains, it rains pennies from heaven. . . ." Lou played the melody on his sax and the organist and guitarist improvised about as slow as a leaf floats on a windless day—moody, dripping with soul. The lyrics of the tune had to be true. Celestina and I would have been lulled by them all the way uptown, if she hadn't spotted the poster.

"Pardon me," Celestina responded calmly to my blunt negative about the walk. She hardly ever veered from serenity, except onstage. She ran her fingers through her shoulder-length blonde hair. "I just thought you might *possibly* want to go— you know, being a survivor."

"I've never given the American Cancer Society a dime and never will!" I sat up, stretching my spine to its full length like an exclamation mark. "Millions have been poured into cancer research from the Society and other organizations since World War II, and where are the cancer cures? What have all those scientists been doing—sitting at their lab counters playing tic-tac-duh?"

Celestina's eyes opened wide. She hadn't yet heard this diatribe of mine, which I'd developed even before my diagnosis. "I really don't think—"

"And why hasn't the Society spent *a lot* more money preventing preventable cancer in the first place? Carcinogenic pesticides in food! Hormones in cows!"

Actually another part of my brain was heartened by recent announcements of "breakthrough" progress in cancer treatment and prevention. But I'd been hearing similar promises for years. Meanwhile, my father's father died at sixty-five of pancreatic cancer; Aunt Ellen, my mother's sister, also died of pancreatic cancer, at sixty-one; and my mother died at seventy-five of lung cancer. I continued my rant. "And why weren't my aunt and mother offered less toxic treatments than chemo? Because these were considered quackeries by the pharmaceutical/medical/American Cancer Society establishment. The American Cancer Scam."

Celestina flipped both hands in the air. "If you say so." She cocked her head. "Consider yourself cast in *Who's Afraid of Virginia Woolf*? You'd make a wicked Virginia." She flicked my hair off my shoulder and whispered, "You could seduce the young husband character with this wild mop of yours and those legs that go on forever."

I bowed my head, delighted by this stroke to my deflated actor ego. I hadn't been auditioning for over three years at this point, and Celestina knew that when I was cast, it was virtually always as a comedienne. She played the gamut from *Noises Off* to *Medea*. I was so proud of her. While I had wandered around Off-, Off-Off-, and Way-Way-Off-Broadway, she had made it to Broadway a few times and had even been cast in a couple of movies.

Celestina looked back at the Cancer Society ad. "I was planning to do the walk—"

"What? Did someone else get diagnosed?"

"No, dingbat, I wanted to do it in honor of *you*."

"Celestina!" I pulled her close and kissed her cheek.

She lowered her head. "I'm sorry—now I can't. I have an extra rehearsal on Sunday."

"I'm so touched you planned to go!"

Celestina continued on the train to the Upper West Side to her third-floor walk-up apartment, while I changed to the shuttle at Times Square and then caught the Lexington north to mine. Finding a seat again, I leaned my head against the metal wall of the car and closed my eyes. "Don't you know each cloud contains. . . ." I smiled, recalling how Celestina had been a sparkling penny when the black cloud of cancer had engulfed me. On tour at the time, doing the séance-loving Madame Arcati in *Blithe Spirit*, a part I drooled for, she'd call almost every day, and she somehow managed to be at the foot of my bed when I woke from surgery. "I felt this tremendous urge, like a rushing wind," she said, borrowing one of Madame's lines, "so I hopped on my bike and here I am."

I had so many gleaming pennies at the hospital. As soon as a nurse showed me to my room, I slid under my pillow a piece of deer bone my brother Pete in Santa Fe had carved into a feather for me, a bar of rose-scented soap from my cousin Kathy in Maine and a St. Christopher medal that my friend Corinne had sent from Paris. Shortly after Celestina kissed me good-bye after the operation, Michael came, bearing a vase of daffodils. Several other friends called. My father, seventy-eight at the time, arthritic, with an unreliable heart and neuropathy in his feet, even made the two-hour trip from Princeton to say hello. My sister Nancy checked me out of the hospital and into her family's spacious co-op on West 107th Street, where she spoiled me for a long weekend with one homemade treat after another, from mouthwatering shrimp risotto to addictive chocolate chip meringues.

A sudden chill in the October night streamed through my trench coat as I exited the subway at Seventy-seventh Street and headed east, but I didn't care. I sang out another line the quartet played: "So-o whe-en you-u hear that thunder, don't, don't, don't run under a tree...." I didn't do that after my diagnosis, did I? Au contraire, I went on the offensive and was now spending over $200 a month on vitamins and no-nonsense supplements like diindolylmethane. I turned up the collar of my coat. Maybe I've been too busy taking care of myself. I've met many breast cancer survivors who are so grateful to be alive and overwhelmed by the support they received, that they devote hours to giving back. I did *try* to give. I started a twelve-step group for cancer survivors in the basement of a Presbyterian church—no one came. I offered a writing workshop for breast cancer survivors at a hospital—nobody signed up. And then there was my stint as an assistant counselor in a cabin of eleven- and twelve-year-old girls, sisters of cancer patients, at Camp Good Days. I hope I helped the girls have a week of fun on the banks of the Keuka, one of the Finger Lakes in central New York State. But the ugly truth is I couldn't wait for the week to be over. I forgot that preadolescent girls in packs squeal. Frequently.

My attempts to give back have been such a bust, and here was Celestina wanting to give even more. I stumbled on a protruding edge of sidewalk. Maybe *I* can improvise a bit: modulate away from who is sponsoring the walk on Sunday and do it in honor of Celestina and everyone else who have been so loving to me.

IT WAS A SUNNY, CRISP, GOLD-orange-red-leafed morning at the Central Park band shell. I leaned against the trunk of a resplendent maple tree and watched waves of women, men and children, in groups of two, three, twenty stream through an arch of pink balloons thirty feet high to begin the five-kilometer walk. Many had writing on their sweatshirts: "NY Chapt of the Legal Secretary's Assn," "Kings County Hospital Center," "I am walking in memory of Sarah," "I Eat Soybeans and Tofu." I cleared my throat, as if this would help me grasp the number of sweatshirts, the number of lives affected by the one-in-eight statistic. More and more waves headed straight to registration tables, handed over cash or a check and strode immediately into the walk—without any celebrity entertainment or even an "On your mark, get set, walk!" This was only the third year the Society was sponsoring the walk in the park, but apparently it had already become routine.

I peeled myself from the tree and started toward registration myself, passing booths hawking Making Strides T-shirts and other Society promotionals.

"Are you a survivor?" a woman called out from behind a table.

"Well, yes." I wasn't wearing my silicone form where my left breast used to be, but how could she detect this through my floppy blue windbreaker?

"Come here." She handed me a bronze medal with "Making Strides Against Breast Cancer—Survivor" on a white decal in the middle. The medal, surprisingly hefty for its two inches in diameter, hung from a loop of wide pink ribbon. "Congratulations!"

I smiled vaguely. "Thank you."

Walking on, I flipped the medal over and over in my palm. A medal for surviving breast cancer? Despite the healthy things I was doing for myself, and my faith in Joseph's regime, I knew that the most fundamental reason I was still alive was ... what? Grace? How could it be grace when so many wonderful people died of this horrible disease? No, it was chance, haphazard chance, just like the second anniversary of my mastectomy landing on Easter.

A medal? The people who deserved a medal were the people who hadn't survived, like my friend Diana, although a lot of good a medal would do them now. I thought of other loved ones who had died—Ma, Daddy, Aunt Ellen and my friend Stu, one of the gentlest people I had ever known, who had been ravaged by AIDS. I would walk for all of them too.

What should I do with the medal? The woman might see if I throw it away. I buried it in my knapsack.

After writing my first ever check to the Society, for $15, the minimum—there was a minimum—I started toward the balloon arch. The musk of fading leaves infused the windless air. I felt as comfy as an acorn in its cup in my favorite old clothes—moth-eaten red sweater, formerly waterproof windbreaker, blue jeans with kneeholes, Nikes frayed perfectly for my bunions. I settled into my usual four-mph New York pace, developed during fifteen years of hoofing it around the city. Smiling volunteers offered bottles of Poland Spring as they directed us and clapped us on. We would do a loop—westward out of the park, north on Central Park West, west on Ninety-sixth Street to Riverside Drive, south and then east on Seventy-second Street back to the band shell. We took over the sidewalk, moving in a collective hush of gratitude for being alive, hope that we would live on, hope that loved ones would live on and bittersweet memories of those we had lost.

Walking up Central Park West, tears swelled in my eyes as I thought of all my friends and family. How could I have lived through the diagnosis and mastectomy without them? Michael, Celestina, Pete in Santa Fe, Jean in Connecticut, Kathy in Maine, who, with her razor sharp mind, helped me navigate the medical and insurance labyrinths—they all seemed to know when to phone. Corinne once called from Paris to say she'd just lit a candle in church for me. I didn't want to forget my former friend Helen, either, who was so sweet to walk me home after my biopsy.

It occurred to me that I still remembered every moment spent with family and friends in the weeks following my operation. My sister took me to see Pavarotti at the Met. There was a flurry of birthday parties. A friend premiered her first film. But my moments with them didn't have to be extraordinary, or, rather, every moment seemed extraordinary—movies, yoga classes, the night three actress friends and I polished off a family-size bag of chocolate chip cookies with a jug of cabernet.

I wanted to honor these dear people by the walk but, as I

strolled along, I didn't feel I was honoring them at all. Really, how could a modest physical activity, one that I enjoyed every day in the city, albeit in other contexts, possibly honor them? It might have been helpful if I'd thought to mention my walking to one of them.

As I was crossing town on Ninety-sixth Street, two women in T-shirts and nylon shorts zipped by—the first runners I'd seen. I winced at them, sure that each boom of their feet on the concrete was assaulting their poor bones. Sympathetic pain shot into my arthritic neck—the main reason I hardly ever ran anymore.

My shoulders started to twitch as I remembered how I used to run in another sense: run from situation to situation to situation, like a squirrel darting about for the perfect acorn, without knowing what the perfect acorn looked like. After leaving my parents' staid, orderly home in Westchester County, I first attended Northwestern, then jumped over to Connecticut College, before dashing to the University of Colorado, where, by some miracle, I graduated. For over ten years afterwards, I jerked about from one career to another—teacher in Cairo, seller of artist supplies on Montmartre in Paris (which position afforded me the occasional baguette), reporter, environmental writer and licensing engineer—never feeling satisfied for long. I was then well into my thirties. One night, humbled by an encounter in my New York apartment, I wrote my first song, "Ode to the New York Cockroach," and I finally began to slow down. Step by step, I wrote other catchy ditties, performed cabaret, wrote a few one-acts, studied acting and at long last began to act. I'd found my acorn! And also, of course, the part-time clerkship at the gastroenterologist's to pay the bills.

When I reached Riverside Drive, I slowed to a stop. I really wanted to run after I was diagnosed, I remembered, run from the frightening evidence that I could die much sooner than anticipated. But how could I run from that? Running wouldn't work at all, especially when I realized that if I did, I might miss something or someone I might not be able to see or hear or hold again.

Oops, I did run pretty much nonstop to find a health plan, didn't I? But I was running like a focused basset hound then, not a flighty squirrel. Right. Totally different.

Proceeding south on the Drive, I was communing dreamily with the glittery ripples of the Hudson River, across Riverside Park to my right, when I almost walked into a foot-high black iron fence in the sidewalk that was protecting a tiny rectangular garden. I knelt down to admire more closely the simple planting of tall, fuzzy pink flowers surrounded by shorter, daisy-like lavender ones. I wished I knew their names but, despite the fact that I had written a double entendre ditty about morning glories and jack-in-the-pulpits for one of my cabaret acts, I couldn't identify practically any flowers. Ma would have found the planting charming, I thought. Dear Ma, I missed her so. She'd loved beauty—irises, the French language, waves crashing against the rocky coast of Maine, Monet. She'd loved to laugh, to sing, to dance on her tiptoes to Louis Armstrong's "What a Wonderful World." She'd loved a number of people, including me. I was sure that her love of life, woven inside me, had helped me to slow down.

Speaking of which, I had slowed to a complete stop again. I was here to walk for my family and friends. I returned to the flow of walkers, still at a total loss as to how the walk could possibly be a tribute to them. What a black-eyed Susan of an idea.

Almost immediately I found myself walking beside a solidly built black woman, also alone, who was ambling along the Drive as though she didn't care if she ever finished the loop. Drawn to her somehow, I adopted her pace. She seemed to be celebrating the season in her pumpkin orange sweats and her earrings—jumbles of black triangles and balls that tinkled with every step. Her mass of neat cornrows was held together by a thin black clasp at the back of her neck. When I offered a smile, she glared at me with tightly drawn ruby lips and quickly turned her head back to the direction we were walking. No doubt about it, she wants to be left alone, I thought. Her face and hands are so smooth, she can't be more than in her mid-thirties, but, Jesus, even though she's not wearing one of those bronze medals, I'm sure she's a survivor. I blundered on. "Your hair is gorgeous!"

"Thank you," she said without looking at me.

"Mind if I ask how many years for you?"

"Two months."

"Oh." My body flashed hot at the shock, the panic she must still be in. I looked over at the young woman again and then in front and back of me at the river of women, men and children walking south. Probably more than one in eight of these women and girls have experienced or will experience that same shock and panic. We are all sisters. With my long, bony hand, I reached for the young woman's hand. I was so glad when hers, smaller and much softer, folded over mine.

Clearly, she didn't want to talk. Plenty of questions came to mind: Are you in treatment? Are you happy with your doctors? Do you want referrals? Do you want my number? Can I have yours? "You're going to be all right," I said.

As we were walking east back to Central Park, our hands loosened, but we stayed close.

By the time we crossed under the arch of balloons again, easy grins had spread across both our faces, and we wrapped our arms around each other.

"Good luck to you," I said.

"You too," she said.

We hugged again, and I watched as she disappeared into the crowd. Good luck, the very best of luck.

Not a bit tired, I began to walk in a big circle around the band shell area, slower and slower, until I was probably outpaced by the drifting leaves. Swarms of others who had finished the walk were also milling about.

At some point I noticed those bronze survivor medals. Woman after woman was wearing one. That was odd—the disks didn't seem silly anymore. They were giant golden eyes, tens and tens of eyes, opened wide, forming a web of caring. They were also brassy proof that breast cancer didn't necessarily mean instant death. There was a lot more life left in all of us. I fished my medal out of my knapsack and slipped the pink ribbon over my head. Count me in.

As I shuffled along again, I began to feel almost dizzy with love—for everyone there and for all the dear people whose faces were flooding my inner eyes, whom I had wanted to honor by the walk, and also for the multitudes upon multitudes of others who were touched by cancer, by other serious disease, by death. Taking in a deep breath, I closed my eyes, and the medals modulated into pennies, so many pennies, floating into me, out of me, filling the air.

Sometimes, as any jazz musician knows, you have to play it real slow.

Rounds, a Friendship in Four Parts

ONE BLUSTERY WINTER AFTERNOON IN LATE 1995, I schlepped down to the West Village to Gilda's Club, a support community for people dealing with cancer that was created in honor of Gilda Radner, the "Saturday Night Live" star who died of ovarian cancer. Gilda's is now in cities throughout the US and abroad.

I had never been to the club before, but my friend Jim, a wonderful poet and actor who was also a brain cancer survivor, had been raving for weeks about a Chinese exercise class he was taking there. I arrived before him and was shown into a large, bright red and yellow room with a circle of stuffed chairs on one side. Feeling awkward without my friend, I didn't even glance at the three women already seated as I settled in. But then I did look. One of the women, the one grinning broadly at me, was Helen. I hadn't seen or heard from her in over three years. What was she doing here?

Lovely Harmonies

I liked Helen's spunk the first time I heard her speak at a women's support group in the West Village one sweltering day in August 1990, almost two years before my mastectomy. "I finally get it," she said. "Anthony was never there for me. I deserve better."

We became good friends, and I was sure we would remain close for the rest of our lives. We had so many things in common. We both wanted to continue living in New York because of our interests in the arts, but only for four days a week so we could spend the rest of our time lolling in some bucolic spot in the Catskills. Unfortunately, neither of us could afford such a lifestyle. Helen, formerly an engineer for the New York Metropolitan Transportation Authority, had taken a modest early retirement so that she could spend her days sculpting. I would be able to afford two homes once I became a fabulously wealthy actress, but in the meantime, I was grubbing along with my part-time gig at the gastroenterologist's.

We both preferred a casual civility, such as enjoying tea and scones while dressed in sweats. We even looked a bit alike, tall ectomorphs with long faces, although no one would mistake one of us for the other since Helen had straight, shiny, naturally blonde hair, while every six weeks I had to dye the insidious white roots of my frizzy tangles back to their proper dark brown. Also, although neither of us was notably gifted at singing (a handicap which hadn't stopped me from performing in cabarets), Helen and I loved to warble together, especially to sing rounds.

> White coral bells upon a slender stalk,
> Lilies of the valley deck my garden walk.
> Oh, how I wish that I might hear them ring.
> That will happen only when the fairies sing.

The most memorable time we sang this sweet one was in the summer of 1991, just after we had arrived at Pumpkin Hollow Farm, a retreat center upstate, south of Albany. With Helen singing one line ahead of me, we repeated it over and over as we strolled over the center's rolling lawns, edged by leafy woods, down to its thriving organic vegetable garden and along a murmuring stream. Blissed out by our lovely harmonies, so easily created, and by the almost magical surroundings, we wouldn't have been surprised if we had heard fairies sing.

We had come to sing our hearts out at a weekend workshop specifically for enthusiastic untrained bellowers. We attended all five of the three-hour sessions, along with some thirty gleeful others, harmonizing our way to heaven on earth through many rounds and easy two- and three-part tunes.

Seemingly mid-song, we found ourselves back in Sir Terry, Helen's rusty brown Ford, returning to the city.

"One of the best things I've ever shared with a friend," I said.

"The best," she said, and then she burst into song. "Thank you for coming."

"Thank you for telling me about it," I sang a third higher.

"Thank you, thank you, thank you!" we sang in duet.

We extended the spirit of the weekend, singing rounds along Manhattan sidewalks, even in the subway to the astonishment of fellow riders, and also at round fests we heard about in the city. One Sunday Helen invited me to sing in the choir of the faded, no-frills Our Lady of Vilnius Lithuanian Church in SoHo, which she attended regularly. Counting Helen and me, the choir consisted of four people singing transliterated Lithuanian to a congregation of maybe twenty people.

Scary Notes

"I'm so afraid I have cancer," Helen gasped on the phone one night that fall.

"What! Why?"

"There's something wrong with my neck. And you know how I walk funny with my left leg?"

"Yes." It was impossible not to notice Helen's pronounced limp. Whenever I had asked about it, she had dismissed my concern.

"Well, I went to an orthopedist today, and he sent me immediately to a neurologist, and I have to have an MRI on Monday!"

"That doesn't mean it's cancer."

"I'm sure it is! My mother died of it, my father *and* my sister." Helen started sobbing.

"What!" Helen had already told me of the deaths of all these people, but she had omitted the causes. I'd never heard of so much cancer in someone's immediate family. I stopped breathing. "What did the neurologist say?"

"He didn't know! That's why he wants the MRI!" More sobbing. "Sorry for yelling."

"Forget it." I had heard Helen snap at people before, and it had always made me uncomfortable. This was the first time she'd aimed her anger at me, but under the circumstances, it was totally understandable.

Thankfully, Helen didn't have cancer, but she did have some weird orthopedic problem that required a delicate neck operation. Surgery went smoothly. I helped her back to her apartment on a quiet block of Perry Street in the West Village, where she would have to remain for weeks. At the time, I was playing Ellen, a palmed-off wife, in Murray Schisgal's farce *Luv* on the Upper West Side, but I saw her in her ground floor one-bedroom when I could, always bearing a large bag of low fat, cheddar cheese popcorn. We'd sit on her living room couch that was pulled out as a bed and, nibbling away, talk, watch a video and sing a round or two.

You haven't been eating scalloped potatoes
For three days, like we have.

We would challenge each other as to who could keep singing, without laughing, this inane dirge-like lament about
Thanksgiving leftovers.

Helen became progressively more sullen. Her doctor directed her not to sculpt for several months, and I was sure this
depressed her, especially since her finished work surrounded
her. Stunning curvaceous pieces up to two feet high in un-
treated oak and walnut sat on various tables and shelves and on
the mantel above the bricked-up fireplace in her living room.
Several more were scattered about on her Oriental rugs.

When she opened the door one afternoon, she was so glum
she wouldn't look up from the floor and didn't even say hello.

"What's wrong?" I asked.

She pointed toward the mantel, to a large mason jar filled
with nuts. "It's from Elaine, a childhood friend from Pitts-
burgh. She has a lot of cancer in her family too."

I tossed my bag of popcorn on the couch bed and rushed
over to read the note tied to the neck of the jar: "Dear Helen,
I've heard from several sources that these bitter almonds prevent cancer. Please eat seven a day. I'm doing it too. Love,
Elaine".

"As if it's possible to prevent the inevitable," Helen mum-
bled, slumping down onto the couch bed. Her hands rested
limply in her lap, fingers up, like snipped off twigs.

"It's not inevitable!" I declared with empty authority.

"My mother had all sorts of odd physical problems like me,
before she got leukemia." Her eyes looked like two blue pan-
sies floating in puddles.

I sank down beside her. "Maybe you should eat them," I

said.

"You've got to be kidding." She grabbed the popcorn bag. "I'd rather stuff myself with this, thank you."

I grabbed the bag back.

She looked at me wide-eyed, and then released her hands to her lap again. "Okay, okay," she said, barely audibly. "For whatever good it does."

I never actually saw Helen eat the almonds, but by December she was her happy, healthy—though still limping—self again. Back at her sculpting, she no longer voiced any cancer fears. Shortly before Christmas, we were invited to a holiday gathering in the Village of people who sight-sang, a cappella, four-part rounds. After imbibing some heavily spiked eggnog, Helen and I took the occasional stab at vocalizing.

Very Scary Notes

Late that winter, the gorgeous Indian doctor found the mammogram of my left breast "highly suspicious" and recommended I have a biopsy ASAP.

Helen was a wonderful comfort to me, waiting at Memorial Sloan-Kettering while I had the procedure and then walking me home. After my surgeon phoned with the bad news the next afternoon, I called her and cried and cried. She didn't say much, but I knew she was listening.

By late the following morning, I wanted to *do* something *with* someone, so I called to ask her if she wanted to have lunch and see a movie.

"Sorry, I don't feel like schlepping uptown today."

"I'll come down to you then."

"Won't that be too much for you?"

"I'll be fine."

There was an awkward pause. "Well, great!" she finally

said. "I'll check the paper for what's playing around here."

When I arrived at her apartment almost an hour later, Helen hadn't put on her makeup yet, so I waited in her living room, admiring her sculptures. "Did you find a movie?" I yelled through the kitchen to her in the bathroom.

"How about *Where Angels Fear to Tread*—2:15 at the Angelica?" she yelled back.

"Perfect!" I'd wanted to see how E. M. Forster's novel translated to the screen.

Helen started singing a wonderful one-word round from Mozart, I followed, and for a couple of minutes the apartment was harmonic nirvana:

Alleluia, alleluia, alleluia, alleluia. . . .

"I really like your sculptures," I yelled after our voices petered out. "They remind me of Henry Moore's."

"A major influence." She laughed.

"I mean it. Were there sculptors in your family in the Ukraine?"

She bolted into the living room. "Lithuania!" she screamed. "My family is from Lithuania! I've told you that. Don't you listen to me?" Her whole face was red. I'd never seen her so angry.

"I'm so sorry, Helen."

She charged to the table behind her couch for a piece of paper, marched over to me and flashed it in my face. "Our Lady of Vilnius Lithuanian Church" was printed in black curlicue type toward the top of the service program. "You even sang there! Lithuanian! Lithuanian!" she yelled.

"I'm so sorry," I repeated. "I don't know why I got mixed up." I tried to make light of my terrible memory, further compromised in this case by my lack of appreciation for Helen's attachment to her family roots. I hardly ever thought about my own British Isles heritage. "You know the Golux?" I ventured. "'I make mistakes but I'm on the side of Good, by accident and happenstance,' from James Thurber's *The Thirteen Clocks*?"

"No!"

We sat, wordless, in our beige booth at a Greek coffee shop, each pecking at our respective egg salads on rye. Finally I broached my suspicion as to why Helen had seemed reticent to see me and had become, I thought, somewhat overly wrought by my stupid "Ukraine."

"It depresses you to be around me because of the cancer, right?"

She continued chewing.

"I understand, Helen. Three people in your family died."

Her lower lip started to quiver.

I leaned against the back of the booth. "I'm not going to die," I declared.

"No," she said in hollow agreement.

"You're not going to either, Helen."

Her face looked drained of blood, resigned.

We walked together down Greenwich Avenue, but when we reached Eighth Street, Helen stopped and clasped her hands. "Guess I'll go. I've got a few errands to run."

"Oh. I'll meet you at the theater then."

"No, I don't think I want to see the movie. But you go."

"What?"

"I've got to go." She gave me a perfunctory hug. "I'll call you."

I stood, frozen, watching her race down Eighth and disappear left at Fifth Avenue. Having no spirit to see the movie alone, I returned home.

The next day I called. Her machine clicked on, so I left a

message. A few days later I left another message. She never called back. I was devastated.

Reprise

Over three years passed without a word, and then Helen was smiling at me from her chair across the circle at Gilda's.

"Oh, hello," I said faintly.

"Hello, Susan!" she said enthusiastically. She walked over. Both her jeans and faded olive green sweatshirt seemed at least two sizes too big for her, and the lines on either side of her mouth and across her forehead had deepened. "Are you a member?"

I stood up and shook my head. "A guest of Jim's."

"Oh, he's marvelous!"

"He is."

She raised her eyebrows and tilted her head. "I've been a member for months."

"You have cancer?"

"A rare kind—of the blood." She was still smiling, perhaps feeling the easy closeness cancer survivors often feel with one another, perhaps happy to see me, perhaps both.

"Oh," was all I was able to say, thus creating a conversational vacuum, which sucked her back into her seat. Jesus, I thought, she really did get the disease she'd dreaded.

Mr. Loo, trim, muscular, maybe forty, maybe sixty, breezed into the room and directed us to stand and form a circle. I carefully positioned myself one person away from Helen, but throughout the class she leaned in front of the short, good-natured woman between us to whisper pointers to me.

"If some day exercise do, some day not do, not good, not bad," Mr. Loo began. "If exercise every day do, is good."

Jim rushed in. He and I smiled hello as he found a spot opposite me in the circle. Mr. Loo led us gently through eight breathing exercises, some "energy" movements, exercises to move the lymph and several more to strengthen the abdominal organs. Helen and I exchanged giggles as Jim threw himself into the movements. Skinny and six foot two, with his long arms and legs pumping and stretching, he resembled a giant insect performing an elaborate mating ritual. Helen was able to do the routines, but without the vigor I'd remembered.

I met up with Jim at the snack table for some naturally decaffeinated green tea, and was about to tell him he'd be a shoo-in for giant praying mantis roles, when Helen joined us already wearing her camel hair coat. "It's so nice to see you again, Susan. I was just thinking this week of that singing weekend at Pumpkin Hollow Farm. You remember?"

"Oh, yes."

"You coming next week?"

"I don't know," I said, still in shock at seeing her.

"I hope you do. I don't remember why we drifted apart."

You don't?

I enjoyed the class but didn't return. My schedule was already very full, and even if it were not, I'd have to face Helen again. Still, I couldn't get her out of my mind, so a few weeks later I called. We talked for almost an hour, cautiously revealing news of ourselves. I couldn't follow all the details of her cancer, but the sad gist was that she had lost twenty pounds, she was getting progressively weaker, and her cancer was incurable. She still couldn't remember why we'd stopped talking.

"Because I mixed up your Lithuania with the Ukraine, but mainly, I think, because I got cancer," I said.

"You're kidding!"

"I've been very upset—the way we just stopped being friends. You never returned my calls."

"I didn't?"

How could she forget that? "No."

"I'm so sorry, Susan."

The sincerity I heard in her words was like an instant muscle relaxant to the knot in my stomach. "It's all right," I said. I sighed. "It's wonderful to be talking with you again. I've missed you."

"You too."

On my way to Gristedes Supermarket later, I even began to hum—softly, so as not to embarrass myself—a round I'd learned back when I was in the Brownies:

> Make new friends but keep the old,
> One is silver and the other gold.

But the rhyme proved overly simplistic. Helen called a few days later to ask if I'd like to see a movie the following evening. "I'm sorry, I'm already busy," I said, surprised at my relief. I never called her again. I knew the warmth of friendship would comfort her now more than ever, but I guess my hurt and distrust of her ran too deep. All I could do was wish her well through the ethers, wish her all possible blessings, and hope she already had plenty of support. She never called me again either. We had both tried to renew our friendship, we did sound it out, but I'm afraid it had already been rounded out, drowned out really, by the cymbal clash of cancer.

> *Dona nobis pacem, pacem. Dona nobis pacem. . . .*
> (Grant us peace, peace. Grant us peace. . . .)

12 ɚɔ

Growing Like Hops

THE FOLLOWING SPRING, MY FRIEND JEAN PHONED from Connecticut full of excitement. She had a new client, Paul, who was going to pay her thirty dollars an hour to take care of his numerous flower gardens. In addition, Paul had hops vines growing in his backyard, and if she tended them, he said, she could sell the hops to the microbrewery he had been supplying and pocket the money. A couple of weeks later, Jean called to report that just as the vines were beginning to sprout, she pruned them back.

"The poor things!" I protested.

"No," she said, "Paul told me to prune them right to the ground to get strong regrowth and good cones."

"Cones?"

"Flowers. I'll sell the dried flowers."

"Oh," I said, not really understanding any of this. But now I realize I had a lot in common with Jean's hops.

Earlier that year, when the soil in the Northeast was still

frozen, I received a mailer from Memorial Sloan-Kettering. The hospital's counseling center was offering current and former patients free art therapy sessions. I registered immediately. I knew nothing about art therapy and my drawing ability was at the stick-figure level, but I had to try it. It had been four years since my mastectomy, and my life was *still* being defined by cancer. Despite following Joseph's pill regime, I continued to get bolts of terror that I would have to face cancer again. I was still sad and also—this infuriated me—ashamed that I was one-breasted. I kept slogging to my clerkship at the gastroenterologist's, without using my free time to audition. I still had no love life. The only times I felt exhilarated were when I was saying my affirmations. Alice, my counselor, kept trying to coax me out of my morass, continually pointing out that various self-defeating beliefs and behaviors weren't part of my DNA, but it was obvious to me that I needed some altogether different kind of help.

Celestina was having a blast analyzing her dreams with a Jungian therapist. I wanted to see him too. Dream images, so different from words, would be indisputable subjective truths straight from my subconscious! Obstacle: I couldn't remember my dreams.

Entering the counseling center's spacious waiting room on Second Avenue, I was worried about my drawing disability, but excited that the sessions would surely deal with images. I hurried down the steep stairs to the basement into a windowless, white-walled conference room. Nine other women were already seated at the long, white laminate table. For more than a year, I would spend two hours a week in this safe, womb-like space.

I drew an image that very first day. The art therapist, Paola, directed us to close our eyes and move our pencils around our sheets of white paper as if the pencils were "taking a walk." After a minute or so, we were to open our eyes and develop our "blind" drawings.

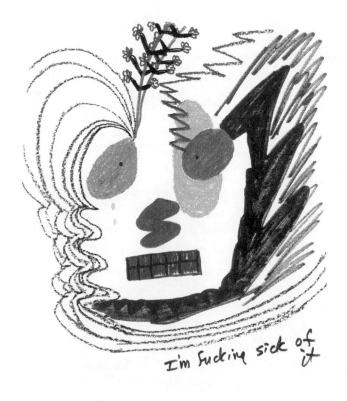

It was a relief to get my feelings out. It was actually joyful to give them shape and color.

We all titled our pieces and then mounted them on a wall with sticky putty. Despite the crudeness of my image, I liked looking at my anger and sadness from a distance. And I wasn't only those feelings. I was also the various lenses, the flowers, the zigzag nose—lighter aspects of myself hard to access since my mastectomy. I felt vibrant, even minimally artistic.

Each woman discussed her work in turn. I found everyone else's unique, striking, beautiful and also comforting since almost all of them were drawn in about the same five-year-old style as my own. Although each piece expressed difficult feelings, nobody had an emotional outburst. No one shed a tear. Our feelings seemed to be contained in our pieces, at least during class.

When I got home, I jotted down a verbal equivalent to my piece (a practice I would continue after most sessions):

Angry, jagged, black on black, teeth red with fury and tears.
Yet, three different lenses to see through—sky blue, tree green,
*   placid pink.*
The elephant trunk of a nose wants to unkink, stretch up and
*   smell the posies.*

The ten of us, ranging in age from twenty to seventy-two, from various walks of life and survivors of different kinds of cancers, would gather around the conference table week after week. We never got to know each other in the everyday sense. Perhaps we wanted to keep our distance from the intense seriousness we shared in the room. But we quickly developed a warm bond in class. Paola made us feel comfortable from the start, always speaking calmly, sparingly, in the musical cadence of her Italian accent. She was like an elfish Buddhist monk, short and slight, with closely cropped salt and pepper hair, always slightly abstract in her black slacks and white doctor jacket. As we worked, she would walk slowly around the table and watch over us, her hazel eyes soft as down, sharp as a mother eagle's.

Paola provided us project after project in which we could experience our psyches as simultaneous universes of darkness and light. In one workshop, she scattered magazines around the conference table and asked us to cut out images we responded to, even if we didn't know why. In the time allotted, maybe twenty minutes, I pasted twenty-eight images onto my eighteen-by-twenty-four-inch sheet—from a man lying on a bed of nails, a woman sitting in a chair with downcast eyes, a boy screaming, to a lackadaisical manatee, a woman offering a ripe artichoke from a field of them, a woman dancing in ecstasy. When everyone displayed their pieces on the wall, I identified with more images—a fierce gargoyle, a man contemplating a dormant geyser, a man singing with so much joy he could have made the whole world smile. Our psyches seemed to be truly bipolar: we wouldn't be able to sing unless we also felt the sting of nails.

One day, Paola scattered magazines around and directed us to cut out words we responded to along with images. On the left side of a piece of paper, I pasted an image of a man shooting a rifle, with the words "dangerous" and "confusing"; on the right side, a long, lush vine and the words "thrive" and "celebrating"; and in the middle, two elephant seals fighting for dominance. I think the words brought the myth-like images closer to my everyday world. It was interesting that the words on the left were adjectives, and those on the right, active verbs.

The next week, I seemed to speak for one of those seals. In a variation of our first session, Paola asked us to make a real mess with tempera paint on our blank paper and then, on other sheets, to expand one or more areas that attracted us.

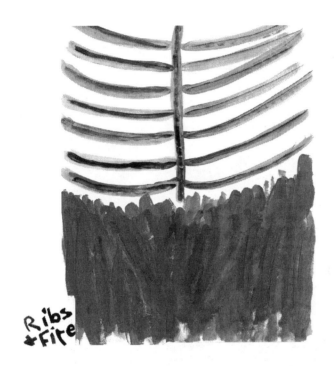

Ribs as strong as black wrought iron,
Ribs as seasoned as rock rubbed smooth,
Ribs as fresh as green leaves in May,
Ribs as light as a fluttering Monarch,
Ribs as proud as orange roof tiles in the Tuscan sun,
With a red-hot fire of a heart that will not be subdued.

Months of art therapy passed, each session nurturing, moving and full of amazing, uplifting discoveries. And yet my fear, sadness and anger about cancer wouldn't go away! One day, furious that I was still boxed in by these feelings, I arrived at the conference room hellbent on using art to banish them once and for all.

As fate would have it, this week Paola asked us to give up practically all control over what we made. We were simply to put blobs of tempera paint on a sheet of paper, place another sheet on top, squish the paint around from the top of the top sheet and then lift off the top sheet to see the result.

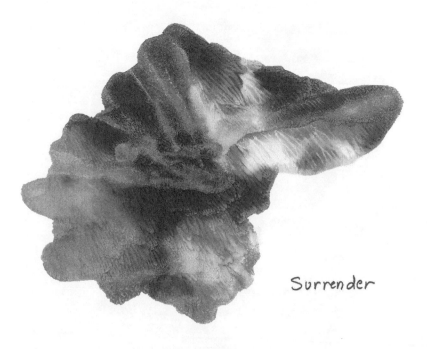

Surrender

The elegant purple-yellow iris floats in on her diaphanous petals, wafting a heavenly scent, and whispers to the livid red face,

"I feel your pain. That's why I came.
It hurts me so—your despair, watching you glare at your life.

I know. I know.
But let it go. Don't you see?
Let it all dissolve in me."

I'd come to the session livid with all that will, and an image I played no conscious part in creating—an image of surrender, of all things—emerged. The tautness in my shoulder muscles relaxed. I felt visited by a powerful benevolence.

That same day we all saw another woman's image, at first, as a beautiful symmetrical abstract design in green, blue, yellow and red. But soon we realized it was suggestive of a woman's vagina surrounded by layers of graceful labial lips and then hips. The room fell silent.

"It's a magic shield," someone finally whispered.

"From a Native American medicine woman," continued someone else.

"It's healing us," a third woman added.

Everyone felt it. Paola, usually reticent about expressing her interpretation of anyone's work, chimed in, "Yes! Yes!"

More months of art therapy passed, with one mind-blowing session after another. And yet outside the conference room, I continued to be the suffering cancer survivor—until a certain phone call pruned me to the ground.

Michael and I were still very close friends. He or I would call at least every other week. "You're a hard act to follow," he would comment during practically every conversation.

Hard, but, it turned out, not impossible. Recently he had become bored with his job as a music and sound effects editor and was increasingly enthusiastic about his new membership in the New York City Sierra Club's photography committee. I was proud of him. Usually shy, he'd never been a joiner before. During this fateful call, he mentioned ever so casually that he had a new girlfriend, someone in the club. "Really? I'm so

happy for you!" I managed, tears flooding my eyes. I faked
that my intercom was buzzing and got off the phone.

Michael's news plunged me into deep despair and self-
loathing, as if he were deserting me, as if I were now definitely too ugly and damaged to ever be a lover, to ever find any
happiness in life. When I went to art therapy the next day,
I chose tempera paints and didn't listen to the activity Paola
suggested.

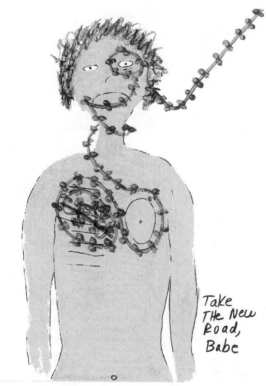

A slash where my breast used to be—red, ugly, ugly.

No man wants me. I don't want me.
Michael and what's-her-name are obsessed by the possibili-

ties of each other while I am obsessed by the possibility of
death.
It is of absolutely no solace that I broke up with him!
Ugly, ugly, ugly.
Fuck!
I now use that word in vain.
Fuck, fuck, fuck!

I stare at the slash on my paper. Why didn't my surgeon slice
deeper, through my heart?
It feels like she did. I zero in, see nothing but the slash.

But then—am I hallucinating?—I see beneath the slash,
something beneath the slash, something green—a green vine.
The vine grows and grows, out of my heart, through my slash.
It twines round and round the slash, around my other breast,
reaches up and garlands my neck. It upturns my frown, encir-
cles one of my eyes, one of my ears, and then grows off the page.

"Take the new road, babe," it says.

Only my brother calls me "babe," like I'm one of his close wom-
an friends and he's too shy to say, "I love you and I want the
best for you."
"Take the new road, babe."

Years later, I realize that drawing this piece changed my life.
I'd made a decision while drawing it, a decision deeply rooted
in months of exploring the shapes and colors of the human
psyche, a decision that finally burst out of me when my life
seemed utterly destroyed. I would take the new road. I didn't
have to dwell on my losses. I didn't need men. I had a lot to
live for without them—wonderful girlfriends, seemingly good

health, things I wanted to do.

I retrieved my silicone breast from the back of one of my drawers and started auditioning. I was still the "red slash," still the cancer survivor, but I was also the "green vine," and, like Jean's hops, I was now determined to reach toward the sun. In a few weeks, I landed the part of Corie's soon-to-be unconventional mother in Neil Simon's *Barefoot in the Park*, in Brooklyn. In October of 1997, I got two callbacks for the plucky Madame Arcati in *Blithe Spirit*. Inexplicably, the director chose another actress, who couldn't be flamboyant if she were dancing the flamenco. Oh well, at least I didn't harbor any resentment about it.

13 ॐ

Blending In

WHAT DO BOTTICELLI'S BREEZY *The Birth of Venus,*
Rodin's exuberant marble *Eternal Spring* and an iconic bronze
statuette of Aphrodite from the first or second century B.C. all
have in common? Each of the nude women depicted has size
A to B breasts. I know because for several weeks in late 1997,
I investigated nudes and partial nudes at the National Gallery
in London and the Metropolitan Museum of Art in New York,
as well as in various art history books. My study began when
I bought a cheap flight to London that November for a "city
break," and I wandered into the National. Almost immediately
I was seized by the notion that I might somehow vanquish my
lingering sorrow and anger over having been reduced by a mastectomy to one breast, which was quite small—one might say
as small as a breast could be and still be a breast—by feasting
my eyes on beautiful depictions of breasts in works of art.

Too often, I felt compelled to estimate the sizes of the
breasts, in an effort to determine if my diminutive right breast

was as rare in days of old as it seemed to be now. The answer, unfortunately, is a flat yes, or at any rate virtually none of the artists seemed to consider AA breasts beautiful enough to depict. They fixated practically exclusively on A to C breasts even without a modern bra to help them measure. Only one painting displayed a pair of breasts that seemed smaller than A—those of Venus in Cranach the Elder's *Cupid Complaining to Venus*, circa 1552, at the National. That was over 450 years ago. Cranach's Venus, I would like to report, looks sensuous, fetching, I dare say elegant.

When I returned to New York, I did come across eight small figurines at the Met with pimple breasts—from ancient Cyprus, Iran and Ecuador (the gender of the Ecuadoran was questionable) as well as the prehistoric Cyclades and the Democratic Republic of the Congo—but these were highly stylized, surely not intended to be realistic. I also saw three of Degas' charming bronze statuettes of dancers who were minimally breasted, though I shouldn't count one of them since she was in a costume, not nude, and, according to the title, the model had been a fourteen-year-old. These were the only depictions of subtle breasts I found.

I even sought professional help to verify my findings.

"Susan, you're not wearing your breast form," Bernice reprimanded as I stepped through the door of her dressing-room-size boutique on the Upper West Side, which was still bursting with bras and panties. I assumed my chest would be impossible to critique underneath my turtleneck, wool pullover and shapeless down coat.

"I know," I said sheepishly, recalling how she had so tactfully fitted me years earlier with the smallest silicone form she'd probably ever sold.

Bernice was au courant as ever in an aubergine pant suit and a flowery gray silk blouse that glamorized her silver hair.

She rushed around the counter to give me a hug.

"It's so sweet of you to remember me!"

"I remember all my girls."

We chatted about some breast cancer survivors we both knew as I unzipped my knapsack on the counter. I bet Bernice remembers all her girls' breast sizes too, I thought. I've come to the right place. "Do you have a minute?" I pulled out a stack of postcard and xeroxed reproductions of nudes and partial nudes, and asked for her help.

"Aha!" She whipped a magnifying glass from under the counter and set straight to work, considering each breast as if Sherlock Holmes required her immediate professional opinion. Her verdict: all my A to C estimates were correct, except that Delilah fatally tempted Samson in Rubens' *Samson and Delilah* with Ds (!) and the *Dancing Celestial*, a sandstone statuette from twelfth-century India, flaunted DDs (!!).

While still in London, after I'd whipped through the National to size up the breasts there, I took a break for lunch across the street at the Café in the Crypt, downstairs in Saint Martin-in-the-Fields. I recommend this calm, dimly lit spot, by the way, where you can eat, listen to Handel on CD and view the tomb of the furniture maker, Thomas Chippendale, all at the same time. I sat at a small table with my tuna on a roll, and proceeded to estimate that the size of the roll was about that of an A breast. Enough with breast size already! I was appalled at myself: I had just spent two hours cruising by beautiful works of art only to quantify, rate, objectify the breasts—behavior for which I had long condemned American men. Of course, men weren't the only ones. I remembered an exhibit I'd seen years earlier in Tribeca, when this area in southern Manhattan was considered très avant garde, in which a woman artist had made plaster casts of ten of her friends' breasts and arranged them by size on a table. I'd found the breasts themselves moving, but the lineup looked about as aesthetic as a shelf of plaster uppers and lowers at a dentist's office.

I nibbled slowly at my tuna roll. I knew I wouldn't be able to stop myself from estimating breast size in works of art. But, I resolved, henceforth I would also take the time to delight in the artistic renderings of the breasts, in the context of the rest of the female body depicted and the whole work.

Returning to the National, I was attracted to paintings that depicted stories. A former English major and an actress, I liked stories. I paused before Tintoretto's *The Origin of the Milky Way*, in which milk is spurting as if from faucets out of a nude's breasts. According to the explanatory plaque, the left breast of versatile Juno, the Roman goddess of women, is aimed upward to birth the Milky Way; her right breast points down to give rise to lilies. My spine stretched up, my ribs puffed out with pride at being a woman, a woman among women—at the life-giving power inside our breasts, at our potential to create, to nurture, to love.

In Rubens' magnificent *Peace and War*, Peace, accompanied by happy followers of Bacchus, the god of wine and fertility, sends forth her abundant breast milk to the infant Plutus, the god of wealth. The joyous, sunlit group is guarded by Minerva, the goddess of wisdom and the arts, who wards off dark Mars, the god of war. I beamed at this celebration of Woman as a sustaining and life-enriching force.

Over the following days, at the National and then in New York, I became entranced by one great painting after another of a full or partial nude that told a tale—more allegories, bacchanals, Bible stories. I appreciated briefly the artistic values of each work—the color, light, lines and shapes—and I admired ever so briefly the sensuousness of the nudes, including their breasts. But my primary involvement was the story. I was used to stories.

I wasn't at all used to looking at female nudes. I'd only been unclothed with other women when we would change in dressing rooms or on overnights, and even then, I would always avert my eyes, terrified that if I glanced at them, they might reciprocate and gawk in disbelief at my limited chest—and ample rear.

Plus there was the Jayne Mansfield factor. I met her when I was twelve and absolutely flat. On a family vacation in California, my father arranged for us to tour a Hollywood studio. We were standing in a hallway with a studio executive when she happened by. "Come here, Jayne," the executive called to her, "meet the Cummings." She was a goddess—tall (she must have been wearing spike heels because I Googled her and she was actually only about five foot six) with porcelain skin, bouncy platinum-blonde hair and a torso of nonstop curves. She was squeezed into a tight tan skirt and an even tighter yellow, deep V-necked sweater—a sweater in August. She seemed delighted to meet us. "Hello," she said, flashing an easy smile. Struck dumb, I couldn't muster a sound. I had never seen, never imagined such swellings. Instantly I knew that I would never look anything remotely like Jayne. I think it was at this moment that I made a definitive life decision: I would concern myself with thinking and with seeing *inner* beauty.

Add to this history the loss of a breast, and you have a woman who, determined to enjoy artwork of nudes, preferred those where the bodies were *doing* something, not just standing or sitting around, demanding that she consider them solely in their corporeal glory.

But then one day at the Met, I was forced to a full stop by a virtually nude Venus—young, fetching, indulgently fleshy. She is lounging indolently on a gilded couch as if she'd just as soon never move again. And why should she, surrounded by opulent drapes, befriended by graceful doves and attended by three adorable Cupids adorning her with pearls? Francois Boucher's

The Toilet of Venus made me feel rich and dainty from head to toe, as if I were about to put on an iridescent powder blue taffeta gown and attend a Paris ball. My eyes never lingered on Venus' partially exposed breasts. The pull of the piece was its *overall* prettiness. Still, I was now able to enjoy certain frilly, as it were, depictions of nudes, whether there was much of a story to them or not.

A few days later, flipping through an art history book, I came upon *La Baigneuse blonde* by Renoir, a painting I had always raced by before. This time I was transfixed. A young nude is simply sitting in three-quarter view, with one arm resting on a thigh, the other effortlessly holding a white sheet that partially covers her legs. While previously my eyes had judged—naughty me—her round, buoyant breasts as way too big, Cs at least, I now found them luscious. Before, I had also been put off by her ample tummy, thighs and hips, but now I found this abundant fleshiness rich, captivating. She was highly sensuous, exquisitely so, with a sweet, open face. I couldn't keep my eyes away from her pale pink-white skin. Aglow from its glow, I wanted to bask nude in the noncarcinogenic sun right beside her. And this was only a five-by-seven-inch reproduction.

I was finally enjoying the very nudeness of nudes—with their bounteous breasts. At the Met again, a graceful Roman statuette of young, slim Aphrodite caught my eye. Lit from above, her marble head and slightly tilted torso were translucent white, except for dark shadows on the lower sides of her breasts, stomach and pubic bone. The statuette brought me to tears—its ineffable perfection, the female body in one of its simplest ideal possibilities. I couldn't see enough nudes now—Titian's *Venus and the Lute Player,* Courbet's *Woman with a Parrot,* striking cone-breasted figures from the Democratic Republic of the Congo, sumptuously bulbous Hindu goddesses from Cambodia.

I wasn't expecting to see any one-breasted women at the Met that day, except perhaps an Amazon or two. I did find one Amazon, a Roman marble, but she was two-breasted—probably a commander. However, much to my surprise, I did come across about thirty paintings and sculptures of women with only one breast exposed. In all these works, the existence of a second breast under the woman's clothing was no doubt understood if not actually indicated. But I was elated to see that the women depicted, the likes of many a Mary breast-feeding baby Jesus, for God's sake, looked beautiful with only one breast showing, that the one breast shown looked beautiful, that one breast was enough.

You might say that all the nudes I viewed during my beautiful breast survey were decidedly not me. Virtually all of them had plump breasts, explicit or implicit pairs of them, every one of which, by the way, triumphed over the force of gravity. They were all also blessed with youth and smooth, cellulite-free skin. But, whatever their endowments, I now looked at them without envy, without feeling inferior. They now filled me with unconditional delight. A rich palette of female nudes had blended its way beneath my skin. I, too, was made of skin and flesh, and skin and flesh were beautiful. All bodies were beautiful. A few wrinkles, a little cellulite—so? Two breasts or one, large breasts or small—all were lovely. If Renoir were to paint me nude, I was sure he would create a most pleasing work.

14 ❧

Becoming a Belle of a Certain Age

Dance Position

ONE MAGIC SPRING NIGHT WHEN I WAS TWELVE, MY family drove to New York to see *My Fair Lady* on Broadway. I sat transfixed as Eliza Doolittle and Henry Higgins, accompanied by an orchestra, funny song by angry, sad, sweet song, fast dance by slow, fell in love. On the drive back to Westchester, I was glad for once to be squished between my older brother and sister in the backseat of our station wagon. Otherwise, I would have keeled over from the splendiferous wonder of it all. Eyes closed, I immediately set high standards for the love of my life: he would have to speak with a foreign accent, and we would have to dance together triumphantly at a ball.

The following summer, I readied myself for my certain future. Crouched in about three feet of water in the lake in front of our summer home in the Adirondacks, I would belt out my favorite number from the show: "I could have danced all night.

. . . " On "danced," on every sustained word, I would jump up to fling my arms and legs wide—my version of a ballerina's leap—before collapsing into the water. No longer a gangly recovering tomboy, I was the star of Little Moose Lake and also, in a parallel reality, a graceful, charming princess who had usurped Eliza and was the belle of an utterly grand, chandelier-lit ball. I was waltzing round and round the marble floor with one dashing partner after another, especially the tall, dark-haired, refined but irreverent and ever-so-British Henry.

My teenage years didn't turn out quite this way. For starters, I didn't know how to ballroom dance. It never occurred to me to take lessons. My closest approximation was at summer dances at Little Moose, two-stepping with blond, blue-eyed Johnny, to whom I was always, unfortunately, just one of many dance partners. I didn't date until college and even then, close to never.

Through the years, as I was busy switching from one career to another, my adolescent standards for love seemed buried deep inside me, like the dead wood in the middle of a tree trunk. I did enjoy liaisons with a few men along the way, one of whom had a charming Israeli accent; another, German; another, Kenyan. But, I note, I never ballroom danced with any of them, and none of these relationships lasted. Then some forty years after my show-stopping leaps in the lake, during three days at the end of 1997, various experiences tapped deeper and deeper into my psyche and drew out that old deadwood, also known as heartwood. Only now my youthful romantic fantasy resurfaced one detail at a time, as real life goals.

By late that December, I didn't have the slightest inclination to ballroom dance or to try to find a man. While I found my one-breasted self worthy of a Renoir, I was sure no man would share my sense of aesthetics, just as years earlier I'd been certain that only I would see my body as a lovely neo-Paul Klee with hieroglyphics. Plus, there was the stigma of having had cancer. But

I didn't care about men anymore. After a year of art therapy, I had stopped affirming à la Louise Hay that I had already found the love of my life—how ridiculous—and embraced the idea that I would live very well on my own.

On Christmas Day, I took the train out to Princeton to be with Marge, now my father's widow for three years. She still lived in their condo. I'd always felt a deep simpatico with Marge. She had lived in New York as a single woman for years, as I was still doing, and we both loved the city and its celebration of the arts. Marge was an aficionada of the New York Philharmonic and art exhibits. She had also enjoyed working in advertising for various agencies, including Compton Advertising, where she had been my father's secretary for years. After my mother and father had separated, when Marge was fifty and my father, sixty, she and Daddy fell in love. They were married for twenty years.

"Sue, Sue, over here!" Marge waved above the crowd on the Princeton Junction platform. Though the light was fading, she was easy to spot—slim, even in her burgundy down coat, her short white hair in soft curls, her face still youthful and fresh with alert blue eyes and smooth cheeks that plumped into an easy smile. She made seventy-three look almost inviting.

Our conversation was wide-ranging, as usual, even more so when Marge's cousin, a gregarious, free-spirited PhD chemist in her late thirties, who was also single, joined us for Christmas dinner. Karen bubbled with excitement about the science fiction novel she was writing and her Shakespeare reading group. The cabernet flowed. Satiated with talk and mutual fondness, and also with Marge's turkey breast with mushroom gravy, mashed sweet potatoes and sautéed asparagus, followed by warm pumpkin pie à la vanilla bean Haagen-Dazs, I couldn't have asked for more. The closest we got to the subject of men was a magazine ad taped to Marge's refrigerator. A bedroom-eyed Adonis was barely wearing a long-sleeved white shirt. "You rogue, you," I said.

Marge arched an eyebrow. "I'll take what I can get."

After Karen left, I went upstairs and wandered into my father's study. Marge had kept the walls exactly as Daddy had left them: covered with framed photos of the two of them at advertising industry events; photos of Daddy with industry people, clients and the likes of Mayor Koch, Presidents Ford and Carter and Queen Elizabeth; and awards he'd received. Amidst these happy reminders of his career, centered above his desk in the largest frame, was a sepia photo of his father.

I only remembered Grandfather vaguely, having seen him last when I was about seven. His photo had never engaged me before. But standing before it now, I felt bathed in his bemused smile, a smile that exuded a warm sense of humor and generous love. Sometimes Daddy had had a wonderful sense of humor too, I thought. Perhaps my father's smile had sometimes resembled Grandfather's. Surely he had known Grandfather's love. In any case, I was suddenly sure that beneath Daddy's disapproval of me, he had loved me. My heart felt lighter, looser.

The following afternoon, bundled in my puffy, green down coat and maroon scarf and mittens, I waited on the Princeton Junction platform for the train back to the city. Initially, I felt a jolly part of the colorfully clad around me—gaggles of giggling teens, couples holding gloved hands, parents tending their tots—all of us making puffy clouds with our exhales, airy accents to the inch of snow that had coated the grass that morning. But then I realized I was the only person traveling alone on the day after Christmas.

I didn't dissolve into self-pity. I was sure I looked the self-sufficient Auntie Mame. But as I jogged in place to keep warm, deep inside I began to feel like a desert in a drought—colorless, dry, empty. A phrase from Peggy Lee began looping in my head. "Is that all there is?"

The next day, I met my friend Celestina in the Village. After lunch we wandered into Loehmann's on Seventh Avenue and gravitated toward the evening dresses. Tucking her shiny blonde hair behind her ears, she held a long, slinky red strapless in front of her and considered herself in a nearby mirror.

"Try it on!" I urged. She would have looked knockout in it.

"Right. Wouldn't it be perfect for lounging on my couch on New Year's, watching a romantic video *alone*?" Celestina's last date, with the incorrigible monologist, had been over two years ago. She walked closer to the mirror and scrutinized the worry lines on her forehead. "I could write a tune on this musical staff."

I moved to her side to examine her. "You need one more line for a staff," I corrected. Considering my own brow, I rubbed the deep furrow that was progressing upward between my eyes. "I have a staff plus a measure line."

This is when the belle-of-the-ball dream began to seep out. With no forethought, I unceremoniously grabbed the red dress from Celestina and swished it in front of me. "Before I have enough measures for an entire song, I'd like to waltz," I said.

Celestina started dancing ministeps in the small space between the racks. "*One*, two, three, *one*, two, three."

"I mean really waltz. And foxtrot—"

"Too stodgy."

"Rumba, samba, tango, the whole ballroom thing. Swing!" She stopped dancing. "You could."

I looked into my friend's brown eyes and whispered, "You know what I've always wanted to do? The Viennese waltz. Wouldn't that be just too much—to be swept around the floor to, you know, *The Blue Danube*?"

"I don't think that's too much," my dear friend said.

She was right. I didn't need to be nubile Eliza or have two breasts or a boyfriend to ballroom dance. I needed dance lessons.

CLAD IN A LONG, BLACK A-LINE skirt, a white silk blouse and, most importantly, a bulky, green wool vest to camouflage my lack of a left breast and my minimalist and unsupported right one, I rode to the fifth floor of a large old brick building on Cooper Square in the East Village. The rickety, industrial-size elevator opened onto a flurry of happy chatter between classes at the Sandra Cameron Dance Center. Almost immediately, a woman announced, "The Basic Six in Studio Three," and ten of us, luckily an equal number of men and women, tagged behind her into a spacious room with a shiny wood floor.

I surreptitiously surveyed the other students. There were no glamour-pusses among us. Good, I didn't want to be distracted. I was there to learn to dance. Suddenly, my inner wallflower panicked: *No one will ask me!* I was obviously the oldest woman there, and, as was often my fate at five feet nine and a half inches, the tallest, even in my flats. A couple of balding men looked even more ancient. They might approach, although one of them was at least half a foot shorter than me. Would I be considered unacceptably decrepit by the slight, fortyish Filipino in the pinstripe suit; the tall, willowy twentyish Japanese; the twentyish blond in black?

I had a short reprieve when our instructor, a young Ginger Rogers in her scoop neck, full-skirted ivory dress, directed us to practice our first slow-slow-quick-quick without a partner. But then Sarah punched in a leisurely foxtrot on the CD player. "Let's try dancing together."

No one will ask me!

Bless her. Sarah directed the men to practice with the woman nearest them and then, rotating counterclockwise, with the next woman and the next—no choosing.

The music made the whole room smile. I enjoyed dancing with all of the men. Each was pleasant and polite, and each kept a respectable distance from my chest. The taller balding man had a balloon of a stomach, but moved with such lightness, the balloon seemed filled with helium. The lanky Japanese led me around with his slender, cool hands like a graceful gazelle. I had to be on my toes, as it were, with the Filipino, who approached dancing like a martial art, strong-arming me this way and that as he punched his feet to the floor like weapons. The other two men weren't always sure where their feet should go, so I pushed and pulled them into place as necessary. They seemed grateful for the help.

The six Tuesday nights glided gaily by as we learned the easiest ways to dance the foxtrot, cha-cha, rumba, tango, swing and—my vision of heaven—the waltz. I and most of my classmates signed up for the next six-week session. I began to apply eye shadow and liner again. My skirts got shorter and shorter. Sometimes, instead of a blousy top, I would wear my enhanced bra and sport a bright, V-necked sweater. I felt prettier and prettier. As the Filipino jujitsued me through the cha-cha one night, he commented, "You look younger every week."

"Thank you," I said casually, as if it weren't the most wonderful compliment I'd received since I couldn't remember when.

I wasn't attracted to him or to any of my partners. I never learned their names, nor did they ask mine. But, while acting ever so blasé about it, I was beside myself, a cat in catnip, having such fun with men, a couple of whom were *less than half my age*. It was downright titillating to hold hands with one of them after another, to feel male arms and hands on my back, to be within inches of male hips and chests. The classroom on Cooper Square became my enchanted sanctuary. While learning my steps, I was also feeling increasingly foxy, without having to worry about finding a man.

But at some point during that second six-week session, the romance and passion insinuated in the music and steps insinuated their way into me, and I got to thinking about dates. I wanted one. I did. What an absolute bummer that I was ineligible.

Change Step

Timing is critical in dancing and also in life. About a week after this upwelling of desire, I found myself sitting in a circle with fifteen other women, including the Memorial Sloan-Kettering social worker who had organized the workshop on, of all things, "Dating and Disclosure."

"I tell dates the scar on my shoulder is from a skiing accident," one woman announced. She looked barely in her twenties, but her low, sultry voice and the short, blunt cut of her pitch-black hair gave her an air of authority.

She got the rest of us to thinking. "I'll say I lost my breast when it got caught in a lawn mower," another woman offered.

"In a Cuisinart," suggested someone else.

"I worked in a kitchen and the chef mistook mine for an onion!"

The group convulsed with laughter.

Most of the women were in their twenties and thirties. Only two of us were old enough to be their mothers. It was heartbreaking to see women so young forced to deal with cancer, but heartwarming to hear them take charge of their love lives.

"Our cancer history is none of their business unless things get serious!" the skier proclaimed at the end of the evening. A silent "Right on!" swept the room.

Right on. I could have a grand time dating men on *my* terms. I didn't have to lie about having had breast cancer, just not mention it. If things got serious—but they wouldn't. I had no interest in meeting that special someone. A special someone spelled undressing. No, no, no. "Girls just wanna have fu-un." I would wear blousy tops or my super bra, and no one would be able to tell. I didn't have to lie about my advanced age either. If a man asked, I'd say dramatically, "I've lived forty-seven years." True. I wasn't thrilled about this slant on my now fifty-three big ones, but was sure it was necessary because, while most men liked to date younger women, I, at this point, had no interest in older men. From my observations, they looked and behaved like senior citizens.

Bypassing the normal hit-or-miss ways of meeting men— I'd missed long enough—I immediately joined two dating clubs that I'd heard about years earlier and filed away: Single Booklovers and Academic Companions. I figured men in these groups would be fairly intelligent and interested in attributes in a woman beyond just the physical. Initial contacts were arranged through the clubs' PO boxes or Academic Companion's new website. For my snail mail address, I provided "c/o Reliable Laundry," conveniently located on the first floor of my apartment building. I don't actually live at Reliable, I would explain to correspondents, but do use it to launder mail.

Both clubs required members to fill out a "profile," from which they would extract a blurb. I felt nude revealing so many details about myself, which I'd normally disclose to a new friend over weeks, months, even years, but reveal I did. I strove to be absolutely honest, other than the necessary omissions of my medical history and part of my age—and, oh, I did lop five pounds off my hundred and thirty, and, well, I did color over the fact that without regular dyeing, my locks would be gray, not brunette, and it seemed irrelevant to mention my ho-hum clerkship at the gastroenterologist's. I said I was an actress and writer currently teaching theater games—all true. I said I loved the city, the country and international travel. I confessed that I was currently in love with Anthony Hopkins as C. S. Lewis in *Shadowlands*, but "might be willing to give him up." I was a somewhat mad recycler. I liked to sing rounds and to move—hike, cross-country ski and most especially waltz. In response to "preferences" I had for a man, I was very open—as long as he was over six feet (I wanted to feel short for a change) and fifty-three or younger, and he lived in the immediate New York City area.

It seemed that no sooner had I mailed my slightly airbrushed version of myself than I received fifteen single-spaced pages from Academic Companions and seventeen from Single Booklovers, all packed with short, tantalizing descriptions of available men—a research psychologist who was also a horticulturalist; a software consultant with predilections for drama and Europe; a children's book editor who liked bird-watching, theater and swing dancing; on and on! I was Belle of the Blurbs.

How could I choose? I crossed out those who were geographically unacceptable. G3571, for example, lived on Long Island. Even that was too far away. Long Island was doubly unacceptable because I'd decided years earlier, based on trips there to visit relatives and friends, that it had deteriorated into irredeemable suburban sprawl. I also x-ed out snobs, like the man looking for a woman of "comparable status;" men who liked to watch baseball or football (boring); men under six feet and over fifty-three, of course; and hyper-intellectuals. One man loved *The New Yorker*, one of my favorite magazines too, but he also claimed to find the time to read every issue of *Harper's*, *The Atlantic Monthly*, *Common Boundary* and *The Utne Reader*. Anyone otherwise acceptable who liked to ballroom dance got two red stars.

After circling twenty male bonbons—five with red stars—I contacted the clubs for their full profiles, and less than a week later, Mei-Lien winked as she handed me two eight-by-ten-inch envelopes across the Reliable counter. I drooled as I climbed the stairs to my apartment. Even allowing for the inevitable airbrushing, practically every man's self-description promised a rich personality, a person passionate about life, someone with whom I would surely enjoy at least an hour's chat.

A few profiles requested photos, so I asked my ex, Michael, with his wonderfully sensitive eye, to snap a roll of me. The photo we chose was beautifully composed, exuding the spirit of Christmas in early spring. I was bright red from my lipstick and earrings to my sweater and jacket, sitting somewhere in midtown with a wall of ivy behind me. Michael and I were sure the photo would be a strong draw. I became even more confident of my prospects when my sweet friend sent me a note clipped to a sample sheet of women's blurbs he had printed out from Academic Companions' website. "I just want to say that you are more than equal to any ad here!"

How many bonbons would I be able to juggle? I contacted the five who ballroom danced—why not go for gold?—sending each a short handwritten note, my profile and a photo, whether they requested one or not.

I received zero responses! How could they all resist that gorgeous photo? Surely my floppy sweater and jacket effectively camouflaged my handicapped chest.

I still have the photo, and now I know how: the men were more interested in the photo's content than its composition, and the content is of a happy, healthy, friendly woman, with a seemingly shapeless, potentially enormous body. It's hard to tell. The sweater and unzipped jacket are both gracefully voluminous.

I didn't initiate any more contacts. I would wait for men in the clubs to choose me.

Some did. In fact, over the next three months, I dated more men, from both in and out of the clubs, than I had in any previous three-month period of my life. Who am I kidding? Three-*year* period. I didn't know what I was looking for in a man. I wanted someone with integrity, surely, and someone with whom I could share an interest, especially ballroom dancing. In the end, I would become surprisingly flexible about a man's height, even age, even geographical whereabouts.

On the other hand, I found a lack of moderation to be a real turnoff. For example, Ed from Soho, who had written me via Academic Companions, was a well-read English teacher and a well-traveled linguist. He sounded worthy of a chat. However, when I had only had time to enjoy a couple of bites of my coq au vin at the West Village café where we met once for lunch, he was already sopping up the last of his pollo con mole with a piece of baguette. I wasn't put off by Ed's size per se—about a third as wide as he was tall—but this, together with an eating speed that surely warranted a Guinness World Record, gave me pause.

If Mark from Queens, a computer consultant I met through Single Booklovers, had been only *moderately* quiet, I might have been interested. His simple, boy-next-door looks reminded me of a fun-loving man I'd acted with in *London Assurance*, a nineteenth-century farce, in a small theater on the Upper West Side. Eric and I had had a blast playing off each other as servants, milking dry our saucy comments during our endless comings and goings. Unfortunately, Mark came up with virtually no lines at our first and only dinner in the Village, just the occasional, flat-toned "Yes" and "No." I had sympathy. Perhaps he had some psychological problem. But it was a chore talking for two.

I didn't think anything of it when another Single Book-lover, Sid, a financial planner from Washington Heights, consumed virtually our entire bottle of chardonnay at our first dinner. Not much of a drinker myself, I was glad he had apparently enjoyed it. But I did think twice when, after a couple more dates, he called to tell me, laughing through his story, how he'd gotten so drunk the night before, he'd had to pull over to the side of the road to sleep it off.

Men appeared where men had never appeared before. I was in menopausal heat. One Sunday, sitting in an oak-paneled room in the West Village, listening to a lecture on Tibetan Buddhism, my eyes listed to the left. Standing by a window, clad in dark chocolate corduroys, a black turtleneck and a brown and black herringbone jacket was a tall, dark-haired man with broad shoulders, an athletic build and a slightly untamed handsomeness to his face. I was drawn to him immediately, I now realize, because of his physical similarity to other important men in my life—my father, my brother and, even after all the intervening years, Rex Harrison as Higgie of London. After the talk, I timed my arrival at the coffee urn to coincide with his.

"Here you go." He offered his styrofoam cupful to me in a *British* accent.

I went to dinner several times with Stanley, an antique dealer originally from London, now from atop the New Jersey Palisades, steep cliffs across the Hudson River from Manhattan. He was beginning to unleash in me tender feelings I hadn't felt in years. But then, one surprisingly sweltering day in May, he picked me up in his shiny red '82 Chevy convertible and drove us down to the New Jersey shore. I understood that we were going there to cool off, but we stepped out of his car for only three minutes at most—the time it took him to buy a bulging basket of clams. He then headed straight back to his condo, plopped his booty on the kitchen counter and, with the aid of a sharp knife, shelled and slurped in one briny, slippery creature after the next. His speed must have qualified him to be yet another Guinness record holder. The empty shells soon formed a mountain in his sink. He continued without a word, without a glance, in a trance. I clammed up. How could he be so immoderate, so un-Higgins, so disgusting? Cast aside for bivalves, I caught the next jitney back to the city.

I couldn't articulate what I wanted in a man, but certain of my chakras knew what got them whirling. One night some girl-friends and I went down to Irving Place, a scruffy dance hall off Union Square, where we'd heard a big band was playing. As we stood on the sidelines, aching to jump and jive to "He's the Boogie Woogie Bugle Boy of Company B," a tall, dark-haired, roughly hewn man in black slacks and a gray and black herring-bone wool jacket—sound familiar?—smiled at me across the crowded floor. I smiled right back. The minute Todor asked me to dance in his deep-toned *Bulgarian* accent, my second-to-lowest chakra started throbbing. It didn't stop for at least a month.

Todor, on the other hand, didn't seem to have a second-to-lowest chakra, or, perhaps more accurately, I didn't turn his on. The aeronautical engineer *claimed* that practically every minute of his waking life was spent in his West Seventy-second Street studio, perfecting his design for the greatest jet engine to ever whiz a plane through the sky. The party pooper never wanted to go dancing again. He could only fit in two-hour visits with me about twice a week, and maddeningly chaste visits they were. Even when I sat beside him at my small kitchen table, thighs brushing, as he played around with my new computer, he never played around with me. Of course, I don't know what I was thinking—I wasn't thinking. I and possibly he would have fainted if he had started something. Somehow I hadn't gotten around to telling him certain anatomical and medical details.

My lower chakra was still moaning for Todor, who was still obsessed with his blasted engine, when I reconnected with an actor I hadn't seen in over ten years, since we'd studied at the Gately-Poole Acting Studio on West Forty-second Street. Our teacher had paired Bill and me together frequently, probably because we were both character actors and about the same age. A wiry man, bright, with a charming southern drawl, he had been excitingly unpredictable as an actor. I had enjoyed working with him, especially in a scene from Tennessee Williams's *The Strangest Kind of Romance*, in which I, a lonely, lusty landlady, tried to seduce him, my extremely reluctant boarder. (I could have played this scene brilliantly with Todor.) When Bill and I weren't rehearsing, though, in his apartment or mine—we both lived in the East Village then—I'd always felt on edge with him because he would hardly talk. Since he was gay, an angry activist, I at first suspected the reason for his silence was that he wanted as little to do with heterosexuals as possible. But then he mentioned several women friends at St. Vincent's Hospital, where he worked in supplies. Maybe he just didn't like me.

Early in the spring of 1998, another actor phoned to tell me that Bill was lying comatose in Beth Israel Hospital. He has been in this state for months, she said, after a truck hit him as he was crossing a street. I went to the hospital several times to talk to him, as many others did, in the faint hope that all our chatter would stimulate him to wake up.

Against all odds, in June, Bill did wake up! He had changed—a lot. His formerly slight body looked even smaller during my first visit after he returned to his tidy studio. His fingers were gnarled, his left leg bent back from the knee, his left foot turned in—all aftermaths of insufficient physical therapy while in the coma. We sat together on a love seat near his two windows facing Second Avenue, the late morning light softened by white lace curtains. Bill loved to talk now. He grew up in a small, Bible-thumping town in Georgia, he told me. Despite this background, or because of it, he became fascinated with Hinduism early on and taught himself Sanskrit. He had been a classical pianist and, even with his current disabilities, he planned to play again. He wanted to know all kinds of things about me. My brush with death and altered body seemed extremely stale news in the telling. We talked and talked. "Life is such a miracle, Susan. Enjoy every second."

We hugged good-bye at the door. His frail body felt as light as a butterfly's. Deeply touched that my formerly distant acting partner had unfurled into a precious new friend, I held Bill closer.

As I say, Bill had changed. "You know, Susan, I'm heterosexual now."

"You're—? "

"I woke up straight."

I loosened my arms and stepped back. "That was some coma." We both laughed. I suddenly didn't know how to be with Bill and left quickly.

My lower chakra finally stopped pining for Todor. I visited Bill many times over the next few weeks. We talked and talked. He became increasingly dear to me. We started to kiss hello and good-bye. I began to imagine us spending longer periods of time together, such as from dinner to breakfast, such as the rest of our lives. I knew I wouldn't be able to do many of my favorite activities with Bill. Ballroom dancing was definitely out. But it seemed much more important to be with this beautiful being, to love him, take care of him. It was as if Bill had lit up my

heart chakra. That re-emerging adolescent image of me waltzing around the dance floor with a tall handsome foreigner was
fading fast.

Right Box Turn

But then through the Internet ethers, I got mail—an email
from Academic Companions with an attached profile of "in-
cog.johannes." Mr. Incog, PhD, was "a successful physicist
working in the medical equipment industry." I liked physics.
He was *Czech* born. I'd always been fascinated by Central
Europe. "My favorite activities include cross country skying,
mountain hiking and ballroom dancing." I loved his spelling
of skiing. And what were the odds of meeting a man who liked
to do three of my favorite pastimes? "I am Bronze 1 level at
Arthur Murray but I am having trouble with the cuddle in the
hustle." The cuddle sounded cozy. This must be a "matchup,"
I thought, a service Academic Companions provided if two
members' profiles seemed compatible.

"I live on Long Island." Ugh. "Age: 59". Damn. "5'11".
Jesus, what was Academic Companions thinking? Did it take
it upon itself to judge that Mr. Incog and I had enough in
common despite his obvious shortcomings?

Of course, I had a few shortcomings myself—not that they
were any of Mr. Incog's business. "Girls just wanna have fu-
un!"

Emails zipped back and forth. I was intrigued. His name
was Jan. How did he pronounce that? "I'm so glad Academic
Companions linked us up," I wrote affably in one message,
still befuddled as to why the club did.

"They didn't link us," Jan responded. "I figured out how to
circumvent the club rules and scrolled through all the wom-

en's profiles until I found you."

Très romantique.

But I was practically committed to Bill.

Four days after Jan's initial email, I met him, at six p.m. on Saturday, July 18, 1998, a sauna of an evening, just outside Central Park at Sixty-first Street. I thought my outfit a good mix of elegant and casual: long, blue cotton skirt that fit to the hips and then flared in soft pleats, with a blousy, short-sleeve cotton top abloom with yellow and blue flowers, which Jean had once informed me were petunias. The top tied at the front, exposing a sliver of midriff. A little exposure never hurt.

I spotted him on the west side of Central Park West, waving a white envelope, our secret-agent method of identity. I waved my envelope back. Watching him cross the street in his neatly creased jeans and short-sleeve plaid shirt, my heart sank. He wasn't just "slim," as his profile claimed, but toothpick skinny. Surely he'd find me, an average "slim," huge in comparison. His light step, fair skin and rimless glasses made him look even more delicate. The closer he came, the more I liked his face, handsome in a Germanic, clean-cut way. I'd have guessed him to be barely fifty. He kept smiling at me. Maybe he didn't mind my size.

"Hi, I'm Jan." He pronounced it "Yan." Sweet.

I never stutter, but I stuttered. "Di-did you have any trou-ble finding this spot?"

"No, I just walked up from Pin Sta-tion."

The conversation was light as we proceeded to Columbus Avenue to find a restaurant. I loved his accent and the way he pronounced every syllable with equal emphasis and distinctly— without slurring or omitting letters the way native English speakers do. I was glad my physical appearance hadn't been his first reason for being interested in me. Surely he couldn't discern what wasn't flowering beneath my swath of petunias, but my hair was as short as a crew cut due to a recent visit to my trendy hairdresser. And with my tendency to drool over big, tall, dark-haired men, it felt healthy and also refreshing that I'd become interested in him before I saw him, and that he turned out to be a very different physical type—slight, about my height, with some, not a lot, of reddish-brown hair.

Over curry at Mughlai, a yuppified Indian restaurant at Sixty-fifth Street, we shared verbal snapshots of our pasts. Jan's, from his life under the Nazis and then the Communists to his experiences in the US, were alternately chilling and in-spiring. He had struggled constantly with the then Czecho-slovakian authorities to be permitted to accept invitations for "scientific stays" in Germany, Austria, Switzerland and even the US. Shortly after the Russians invaded the then Czecho-slovakia in 1968, for example, the government did allow him to work at a physics institute in West Germany, and to bring his wife (*wife!*) and two small children along. But two years later, the government demanded they return home. In 1979, he was even permitted to work at the Brookhaven National Laboratory on Long Island, but only for one year. In 1982, fed up with dealing with authoritarian regimes, he defected to America with his by then teenage son. His daughter joined him a few years later. He still hadn't accounted for *the wife*.

My coddled life seemed too boring to mention—a carefree childhood in suburbia, work in various US cities, except for brief stints in the Middle East and Europe—but Jan smiled at-tentively through every word. I was in awe of his guts to escape at the age of forty-three and also of his achievements here. He worked for an MRI manufacturer, where he was a department head and director of "radio frequency technology"—"It has to do with electric coils," he tactfully dumbed down for me. He had been a homeowner for fourteen years and had put both his children through college.

I was also in awe of the eyes behind those glasses of his.

Small, they seemed to come from deep inside him, as if he only related to things and people at a deep level. But what about the *wife*? I finally asked.

His eyes widened. "I didn't tell you?"

I shook my head.

"She didn't want to move here, our phone calls got more and more argumentative, and we divorced long distance."

Yes!

Too soon he had to race to the subway to catch the 10:39 train back to Long Island.

The following Saturday, we danced the sultry summer night away to a big band in Central Park, inhaling the fragrance of freshly mowed grass, surrounded by the billowy silhouettes of grand old trees and, farther away, the sparkling lights of high rises. I could follow his lead easily. "You're a beauty," he said. I was glad I'd worn my enhanced bra because upon occasion our chests made brief contact, not that we acknowledged this, of course.

Bill called. He asked me to dinner the next Saturday. With the aid of a cane, he could walk to an excellent Italian restaurant at the end of his block.

"Oh, I'd love to, Bill, but I'm going out to Long Island."

He laughed. "I thought you hated Long Island."

"I did, I do," I said awkwardly.

Bill laughed again. "Sometime next week then?" He expected me to suggest an alternative time. I always had when I hadn't been able to see him.

"That would be lovely."

He must have guessed correctly why I was vague. He never called again. I phoned him a few times. I wanted to know how he was doing, to be friends, always friends, but he wasn't interested. He became as distant as my acting partner of years ago. My heart ached when I thought about him. I did want to be with him, to help him, but—oh, dear—Jan seemed to get all my chakras humming.

Jan and I made goo-goo eyes at each other that next Saturday as he introduced me to the beauty and delights of summer in his area of the north shore of Long Island. He picked me up at the Long Island Railroad (LIRR) stop at Port Jefferson Station in his sporty, dark green Honda Prelude. First we breezed past a few soul-numbing mini-malls and McMansion developments, but soon there were fields alive with peppers, tomatoes and corn, and orchards heavy with peaches, on our way to Wildwood Park. A short walk through a green cathedral of woods brought us to an impossibly white, sun-drenched beach and Long Island Sound. Glassy turquoise in the shallows, the water melded into navy blue further out, with a hazy hint of Connecticut beyond. Finding a deserted stretch of sand, we changed into our swimming suits—behind separate black rocks. "You're a beauty," Jan said again when I emerged. I did feel like Jayne M's sister in my electric blue one-piece with its generously reinforced chest. Jan looked ooh-la-la, all pale skin and bone, in his skimpy black Speedo. We dashed in, splashed each other, squealed like kids.

Things were going swimmingly. For dinner, Jan drove us to his favorite Mexican restaurant. Candlelight bathed every table, casting arcs of warmth on the pink walls, which were festooned with huge, colorful sombreros. We were soon savoring a pitcher of cerveza and enchiladas de pollo, but mostly each other. Jan was now the cutest man I'd ever seen. His hands were driving me wild. They were solid, almost square, yet he gestured with them as delicately as a sleepy kitten would a paw. With my chakras ablaze, my little secrets seemed almost trivial, but, still, barriers to closeness. I told Jan my real age. He didn't flinch. I was about to tell him my other significant reserved truth when he brought up the topic of former relationships. Okay. He began to talk specifically about

Linda from Queens. Okay. The first year they were together, he said, he found a lump in her left breast. Not okay! She had a mastectomy and chemo, he went on, but two years later the cancer reappeared, metastasized, and in a few months she died. Not okay! Not okay!

Fork in midair, I froze. Exactly what were the odds of me meeting a man who had been so painfully close to breast cancer? I waited for all the sombreros to fall off the walls and for the table candles to explode. Surely Jan would run the minute I told him what Linda and I had in common. "I'm sorry," I heard myself say. "That must have been awful for you."

"Yes. But that was three years ago now. I am over it."

I quickly changed the subject. Jan knew I was leaving in a few days for a two-week walking holiday in Tuscany. "Would you like me to bring you anything from Italy?"

"Just you."

Molto romantico.

As the train back to New York approached the Port Jefferson Station platform, he kissed my lips for the first time. His felt as soft and plump as baby's skin. Electric shocks shot down to my toes.

Waving good-bye through the LIRR window, I was sure that if he had kissed me or even touched me anywhere one more time, my body would have exploded all over him. I really, really liked him. It was lust, yes, hooray for lust, but I also had great respect for him, already a deep fondness, and I felt such happy, easy comfort in his companionship. *How could I possibly tell him my cancer history, after Linda?*

TUSCANY WAS A FEAST FOR THE senses. Under warm, cloudless skies, our amiable group of twenty, mostly Brits, walked up and down undulating hills, along ancient roads cobbled with history, passing orchards of ripening olives and trellises of swelling grapes. Every four-course dinner included fresh al dente pasta with some delectable sauce. *Il vino* flowed. *L'italiano*, of which I understood the occasional word, was *la passione* set to *la musica*. I'd intended to luxuriate in all this sensual pleasure, but soon I ached to share it too, namely with Jan. *What man would willingly be anywhere near cancer a second time?*

I RETURNED TO NEW YORK ON a Friday and the next day took the train out to see him. Air conditioning was staving off the late August heat in the train car, but my body was still slick with sweat. How would I tell him? I unstuck my pink cotton shorts from the seat and fluffed out my sleeveless pink cotton blouse, rearranging the tissues I'd stuffed into the left breast pocket. I had to tell him. Maybe I could suggest we go to an art gallery. In front of just the right painting, I could ask, "Are you into asymmetry?"

I kicked the heel of my right sneaker into the backrest of the empty seat in front of me. Kick, kick! I refuse to be embarrassed any more that I had cancer! Embarrassed? I'm so grateful to be alive! If he rejects me, to hell with the jerk.

Gazing out the window, my eyes glazed over. He's not a jerk—one in a million is more like it. My eyes closed and I let myself be lulled by the da-da, da-da, da-da sound of the train moving along the tracks—predictable, reliable. I repeated affirmations to myself:

I am beautiful inside and out.
I am perfect just the way I am.
I am loveable and loved and loving.

Da-da, da-da, da-da.
"Port Jefferson Station," the PA system announced.
Jan was at the bottom of the platform stairs in his short-

sleeve plaid shirt and jeans, smiling broadly. My heart leapt.

"Welcome back!" He hugged me and kissed me on the lips.

Electric shocks shot through me just like before. And this was only the beginning of our date. Clothes might very well come off today. *I have to tell him!*

"You want to take a walk on the beach?"

"Sounds lovely."

We settled into his Honda.

"There's something I need to tell you," I said.

"Yes?"

"I'll tell you later."

"Okay." He didn't seem concerned.

This time we drove to the south shore of Long Island, where we crossed a bridge over the Great South Bay to Smith Point on the eastern end of Fire Island. It was late afternoon. People were leaving as we arrived. Even as the sun was lowering and the Atlantic offered a slight breeze, the air was still wavy with heat.

We walked along the white sand just far enough away from the water so the tops of our sneakers wouldn't get wet. Unable to say what I needed to say, I hardly spoke.

Jan began doing 360-degree pivot turns down the beach. "I've learned some new steps in the foxtrot I want to show you."

"Great," I said flatly, unable to muster enthusiasm.

Using me as his spot, he pivoted back toward me, straining his neck to keep his eyes glued to mine as long as possible before swinging around on his foot. I found this effort so darling, I thought my heart would pop out of my chest. Then the possibility that he would reject me made me dizzy, and I stopped, holding my hands to my temples.

"Is something the matter, Susan?"

"No." I focused on the gentle waves—roll in, break, roll in, break. Reliable. Predictable.

We walked back along the beach and sat on a bench overlooking the sea. The sky was turning pink and purple in the west, but in the east was as gray as the ocean.

"I have something to tell you."

"Yes. Okay."

"I'm going to tell you."

"Tell me, please, tell me."

I fixed my eyes on the waves. "I had a mastectomy."

He sighed explosively as if he'd been holding his breath. "Is that all?"

I looked at him with wide eyes. "What do you mean?"

"I knew the moment I met you," he said almost dismissively, as if I'd asked something overly obvious, like the color of his blue-gray eyes.

"What?"

"I've wondered why you haven't talked about it."

"How did you know?"

"I could tell by your blouse."

"But I wore a blousy blouse."

"I could just tell."

"Jesus! Why didn't you say something?"

"I tried. I told you about Linda—"

"I *couldn't* tell you after I heard about her!"

We both looked out at the placid sea. Whitecaps broke in all directions in my head. I finally said barely audibly, "I'm a six-year survivor. Very different from Linda."

"Six years—that's great!"

"So what do you think?"

"About?"

"That I've had breast cancer."

"I don't think about it."

"Come on."

"Look, breast cancer is very common. I like you, Susan. You have so many other qualities. We have so much we can share."

He was one in two million. The waves lapped like soft smiles on the beach. "Thank you," they seemed to say for me. "Thank you, thank you."

JAN AND I SAW EACH OTHER every weekend through the fall, winter and spring. The following summer, I moved into his modern, cedar-sided colonial nestled in pines and oaks. We were giddy non-newlyweds. We could finally take dance lessons together, twice a week at Arthur Murray in a strip mall in Port Jefferson Station. One night our instructor, Daniel, mentioned that in a couple of months the studio would host a "ball," a fancy party where students would perform for each other. A ball!

"What dance would you like to do?" Daniel asked.

"The Viennese Waltz, to *The Blue Danube*," I blurted.

"Sounds good," Jan said.

Daniel warned that the Viennese was not for beginners. "It's fast," he said, "and if you make a wrong move, you could break something."

Jan and I were definitely beginners, but I insisted. Daniel found us a somewhat slower piece to dance to, a lyrical rendering of the theme music from the movie *Papillon*. Decidedly Muzak, it was still charming, featuring an accordion that suggested the venue of a small Parisian café. (Fortunately, Jan and I hadn't seen *Papillon*, the venues of which, I have since learned, are grim penal colonies in French Guiana.) The routine Daniel developed was way beyond our level of incompetence, but Jan and I practiced tenaciously morning and night around the lally columns in his musty basement. We would trip over our own and each other's feet. We would master a step, forget it, swear. "From the top."

"We could pretend we are sick," Jan once suggested.

The big night arrived. Little square tables, each with a starched white tablecloth and the glow of a votive candle, surrounded the dance floor of the studio. Most of the students were in a party mood, joking and laughing. Jan and I, on the other hand, were speechless, terrified we'd flub our routine. He looked handsome, sophisticated and at the same time absolutely adorable in his black tux. I worried that my stomach stuck out in my spaghetti strap, navy blue A-line, but was grateful my reinforced strapless bra didn't seem to be slipping south. We joined a couple we knew at their table, but could contribute only nods to the conversation.

The wall lights dimmed. The dancing began. One couple did a bebopping swing, another steamed through a rumba. There were two smooth foxtrots. Unfortunately, Jan and I were unable to enjoy any of it, being on full *Papillon* alert.

Our turn finally came. We got into position, with me about eight feet to Jan's left. As the introductory accordion and violins of *Papillon* streamed through the speakers, I pivot-turned twice, ending up in front of Jan in dance position, and off we went—left box turn, closed hesitations, change step, parallel hesitations, right box turn. The tiny mirrors of the rotating disco ball lit our way like the Milky Way as we spun around the floor—Arthur Murray turn, promenade hesitations, pregnant pause . . . and then promenade développé (yes, I remembered to lift my leg!), parallel right turns, run and box, spiral turn for the deep-dip ending.

It was over in a twinkle.

The applause was thunderous—enthusiastic anyway. Jan and I squeezed hands as we bowed. We did it, with more flair than we'd rehearsed, with all our limbs intact! I smiled from ear to ear at my marvelous man. A twelve-year-old's dream had led the way. A twelve-year-old's dream had come true—a ball in a mall, but I'd take what I could get.

The Hold of Antiques

DESPITE HAVING JUST REACHED THE SUPERANNUATED age of fifty-five, I was feeling quite the opposite of an antique in the fall of 1999. Jan and I became engaged shortly after the ball. Living with him was still like exploring a new, enchanted country—with a new language. "I'll bet you a kiss anywhere that...." We were still adjusting to each other's ways. For example, Jan was used to vacuuming and dusting, in that order, every week or so, whereas I got around to these activities, in the opposite order, once a quarter, maybe. My New York apartment, comparable in size to below deck in a small sloop, had been furnished in grad-student-grade polyurethaned pine and had looked out through a barred window onto an airshaft. Therefore, I was still either tiptoeing in awe or fast walking for exercise through Jan's spacious four-bedroom *house*, with a first floor *and* a second *and* a basement. It was tastefully furnished with American traditional, and I often felt I was in an art gallery with its walls filled with stunning impressionistic landscapes by his daughter and its tables and shelves with exquisite Raku pots by his son-in-law. Innumerable unbarred windows looked out onto two acres of pristine woods.

I'd bought a car and was still trying to find my way around Suffolk County. "The roads go basically north-south and east-west, so you can't get lost," Jan said. Oh, but I could. To reach Manhattan, where I continued to keep up with various commitments and friends, I would drive my "previously owned" Toyota Corolla from Jan's house west to Ronkonkoma, where I'd catch the LIRR to Penn Station. Normally this drive took about twenty minutes via the local racetrack, aka the Long Island Expressway (LIE).

One October night, however, the drive home took a white-knuckled ninety minutes. Gusts of wind forty-five miles an hour dashed columns of rain every which way against the car. I couldn't decipher the solid line designating the LIE shoulder or the dashed line separating my right lane from the middle one. Heart in throat, I crept along. I tried to laugh: I had now survived cancer for seven years, and I was about to die in a crack-up. Plus, in those seven years, having convinced myself that to prepare in any way for my demise would be to draw death near, I hadn't done any end of life planning, hadn't even called a lawyer to draw up a will.

Inch by harrowing inch, I finally pulled into Jan's driveway, and collapsed over the steering wheel. Thank you, God, luck, hands, alert traffic angels. May everyone get home safely. Gales of rain continued to smash against the car, but from my vastly improved vantage point, they now seemed magnificent, Wagnerian. However, lest I conveniently dismiss what the harrowing drive made clear—that I could die any second—I pushed myself away from the steering wheel and flung open the door. I had to be responsible, especially now with Jan in my life. I would finally deal with my death issues.

Bursting with intent a couple of mornings later, a cloudless, bracing Saturday, I was the first customer at the Wading River Nursery. I would spend the mornings of the weekend creating my first ever garden, near the road to the right of Jan's driveway, and devote both afternoons to making a great start on those funereal matters. Alternating between plants and death seemed a good balance. After lengthy consultations with the nursery staff, I squeezed onto my cart nine daylilies, seven bearded irises, three astilbes and five salvias, all half price because they looked half dead, plus a gold thread cypress, a mix of thirty daffodil bulbs and three bags of composted cow manure. A woman also insisted I buy little sticks to mark where I planted the bulbs.

"Why?"

"Trust me."

A slight breeze blew curled-up brown oak leaves along the asphalt street. They scuttled along like crabs. All focus and connection, I yanked up the grass with a garden fork, dug into and amended the soil and positioned each plant and bulb by whim, confident they'd land where they belonged. Another plant, another bulb, a good watering—somehow I didn't make it inside until dusk.

Early Sunday, a cold and drizzly day, I raced outside to admire my splendid herbaceous artistry before getting down to a whole productive day of death details. No, no, no. I couldn't put my dirty fingernails on it, but the garden wasn't right. How could I sit at my desk knowing that?

Lucky me, I had used the sticks. I dug up and repositioned all my vegetal charges, some twice, some three times, sloshing around in the mud, which eventually slathered my jeans, parka, cheeks and hair.

Jan, much too fastidious to garden in the rain, stepped out at some point to survey my endeavors. "Looking good," he said supportively from under his stately, black umbrella. He seemed quite the country gentleman in his creased jeans, suede slippers and a blue and black argyle sweater that drew out the blue in his eyes.

"You think?"

"Very impressive." He blew me a kiss before starting back to the house, but then he stopped. "You like to dig, don't you?"

"I think so."

"I'm trying to figure what kind of rodent you must have been in your past life."

We both laughed. Jan didn't believe in reincarnation. But he accepted that I did. And I accepted that he didn't. More than accepted—I think we felt expanded by our differences, completed by them.

Just before dark, I managed to unbend my knees and step back to admire what was now sure to be a wondrous garden arrangement. What? I had somehow created a *symmetrical* garden, an almost perfectly *symmetrical* garden. I, who had vowed after my mastectomy never to create anything symmetrical. Symmetry: predictable and boring. Asymmetry: interesting, challenging. I had violated my vow, and also managed to avoid death planning yet again!

After a shower, I stomped into my study—one of Jan's former bedrooms—and, as if they were the problem, scowled at my two desks. One, a door on stilts, was cleared except for a drift of pages from a magazine piece I'd been editing. The other, a lovely cherry wood antique by Chippendale, had its slant-top pulled down as a writing surface. The surface was stacked with piles of confusion—journal notebooks, unpaid bills, unanswered letters, newspaper articles I had clipped and would file if I could decide how to label the files, notes of things to do and remember on bits torn from spiral notebooks, paper bags, napkins.

I plopped my derriere into the office chair in front of the cherry desk. I'd inherited the desk from my mother. Unfortunately, the messy stacks had formed almost immediately after Jan and I had taken it out of storage. I'd wanted to have the desk with me after Ma died, but I couldn't fit it into my crowded New York apartment. I was so glad to have it with me now—something of Ma's. Something of mine—all the furniture in my apartment had been trucked away, reluctantly, by Goodwill.

The house was quiet. Jan was down in the living room devouring the Sunday *New York Times*.

I took a deep breath and retrieved a spiral notebook and pen from the piles. I *will* do my will. I had a little savings. Whom should I give it to? I jotted down Jan, some relatives and friends, some nonprofits—The Nature Conservancy, Planned Parenthood, Amnesty International. What percentages should I give to each? I didn't have a clue. What should I do about my belongings? I had some things others might want, didn't I? Very few, really. Maybe just the desk. I dropped the pen in defeat.

I had to do something constructive. It was Sunday evening, but the local funeral home couldn't be a nine-to-five operation. A bass voice gave me slow, mellifluous encouragement on the phone. "It would be very considerate of you to make preliminary arrangements." Someone could meet me at the home the very next morning.

The Fairmont Funeral Home was a quaint, white clapboard building. Clarissa, Rubenesque, with a creamy teenager complexion, greeted me at the parking lot door. Her somber black-rimmed glasses and tailored, brown corduroy pant suit couldn't mute her youthful exuberance. "Hello, Ms. Cummings! May I call you Susan? So nice to meet you! Come in, come in!"

She was so delighted to see me, I wondered if she might be some friend's daughter whom I'd never met. She led me into her dark, wood-paneled office, where we sat on either side of a huge wooden box of a desk that resembled a coffin for, say, a three-hundred pounder.

I explained that I was trying to get my affairs in order. "I'm engaged now and I think—"

"How exciting!" Clarissa sighed. "I was married once."

"What? Aren't you playing hooky from high school?"

"I'm twenty-six. I've got a six-year-old son."

"No way."

"I wrote a poem about him last night."

"You like to write?"

"Do you?"

I smiled. I'd been focusing more on writing than acting for months now.

Her face lit up. "Want to start a writers' group?"

The invitation seemed a tad hasty. But I'd been hoping to find such a group on Long Island, been wanting to make new friends here too. And, certain that one of the two doors to my left led to an embalming room, I couldn't think of a better time to start. "Let's!"

We chatted for three hours. I couldn't remember when I'd been with someone so excited about life. At noon, Clarissa ordered in two slices of pizza with everything. When the teenager delivered them, I worried that the mélange of smells might be disrespectful, that they might, for instance, waft into some viewing room. But Clarissa didn't seem the least concerned. She took an appreciative whiff of her slice. "Umm. They sprinkled on twice as much garlic today."

We did find a few moments for business. I picked out the least offensive memorial and thank-you cards, both with the same photo of two pines *symmetrically* framing a sunrise.

At some point I noticed a cabinet two feet to my right that was filled with what looked like metal and marble flower vases. That's strange, I thought. Did the Fairmont Funeral Home sell them on the side?

Clarissa saw me staring. "Urns for cremation ashes."

"Right!" I said brightly, as if I were delighted to recall that I had seen one before—my mother's.

"Do you want to choose one now?"

"No, no, I want to be buried whole."

"Uh-huh." She peered confidentially over the top of her glasses. "You might consider cremation. It's hundreds, sometimes thousands cheaper."

"No, not me." That was admirable—a funeral director recommending how to cut costs—but I'd known for years that I wanted to be fodder for the woods. After the tons of food and things I would have consumed during my life, I figured the least I could do was provide a little nourishment for plants and animals.

She looked at me quizzically. "Do you need a cemetery plot?"

"No." I wasn't ready to discuss my fodder plan with her. "I'll have to get back to you on this."

Actually, I did have a plot, my mother's family's plot in Woodlawn Cemetery in the Bronx, but I had no intention of using it. I never even visited Ma there after her funeral. Why would I? I knew her spirit wasn't there. A couple of months after she died, I was walking along Forty-second Street after an audition for Christopher Durang's *The Marriage of Bette and Boo* when she appeared on my left shoulder, an ecstatically happy angel about eight inches high with wings aflutter. My eyes didn't see her, but I knew she was there. Ma! Our hearts embraced. And then she was gone. When I arrived home, there was a message on my answering machine from the director offering me the role I wanted—Soot, a good-natured, somewhat mentally-challenged soul who has her ways of coping with her rat of a husband. Ma must have whispered my praises to the director. She certainly didn't have time for graveyards.

Clarissa and I resumed our happy talk.

"If you think of anything special you want to include in your memorial service, just call. And call about the writing group."

We hugged at the door. Walking to my car, I felt as bubbly as a glass of champagne. Funeral homes were fun.

By the time I reached the post office to mail an unsolicited piece to a magazine, I was smiling so broadly, my lips must have looked like a stretched-out rubber band.

"What's making you such a happy camper today?" the affable counter clerk asked.

I didn't feel I knew Jean Ann well enough to tell her the reason: details of my memorial service. They kept popping into my head. I wanted pots and pots of daffodils. Everyone would sing "Dona Nobis Pacem" as a round, and "The Hills Are Alive with the Sound of Music." My bro Pete would play blues on his harmonica. Celestina would recite Gerard Manley Hopkins' "God's Grandeur," the first poem I loved. Everyone would chant "Jaya Jaya Shiva Shambho" very slowly at first and gradually faster and faster to an ecstatic frenzy. They'd dance to ABBA, the Beatles and Dixieland, Jan's favorite music, and holding hands, yes, *hands*, they'd all dance together in a long line weaving through itself to the Moody Blues' "Morning: Another Morning." There would be gallons of wine; slices of baguette topped with triple crème cheeses, smoked salmon and caviar for Jan; a few token broccoli rosettes; and chewy chocolate chip cookies shaped like hearts. What a party! I wanted to go.

Back in my car again, I even began to warm up to Clarissa's

idea of cremation—the mystery, the momentary majesty, of my body being transformed into the elemental force of fire. And then my ashes could be scattered in the woods.

Damn, euphoria never lasts. Driving home, one thorny funereal problem after another occurred to me: How would the organ donor network learn I was dead? Should there be a little ceremony at the crematorium (or was it a crematory)? Where would the memorial service be? Other patrons of the Fairmont Funeral Home, not to mention its short-term boarders, might not care for ABBA. Where would everyone from out of town stay? How would it all work out without me around to supervise?

I made a U-turn and headed to Super Waldbaum's. I had to discuss everything with Jan, and to ease the way, I'd make one of his favorite dinners, salmon-chickpea-vegetable curry.

"This may sound like I'm getting a bit ahead of myself," I began, plopping a dollop of yogurt on my plate, "but I'd like to be cremated and then disposed of in the woods in back of the house—sprinkled around like a soil amendment."

His shiny eyes fixed on me until he'd finished chewing. "I can't stand the thought of animals eating me. I want to be burned up too."

"We're so compatible."

"But I want a symbol that I made it to America, that I married you."

Oh, no, my Czech-born fiancé wanted his ashes in a cemetery, under a joint tombstone. "Uh-huh." I swished a few chickpeas back and forth.

"Could we be buried next to your mother? Isn't that a family plot?" I must have mentioned the plot at some point.

"It's so inconvenient."

"It's your family."

"My mother's family." I suddenly felt pangs of guilt that I

had never inquired about the possibility of being buried near my father in his family's plot in Illinois. But then, I couldn't imagine Daddy hanging out at his grave either. I most definitely couldn't imagine myself hanging out at mine. How could I acquiesce to Jan on this? I didn't have the stomach to discuss it further.

After dinner I returned to my study and, determined to at least complete my will, ruffled through the piles on Ma's desk to find a notebook and pen. An article I'd clipped about the sex life of sea horses surfaced: Should I file it under "Sex" or "Sea Horses"? See what I mean? I continued my search. Why did I leave Ma's desk such a mess? I hadn't been this disorganized in New York.

Finally I flipped the slant-top up, closing all the chaos in on itself, and then I knew why. My messy piles were best accommodated with the slant-top down, and in this position, the beauty of the desk, which reminded me of Ma, had been largely obscured. Seeing the beauty had been wrenching when Jan and I first placed the desk in the room. But I had been living with it for weeks. Now its beauty seemed tender, joyful. It was as if Ma's soul—something like the air at the edge of a pond bordered by flowering dogwoods—had floated out of the wood and enveloped me.

I ran my fingers along the grooves of the large scallop shell design carved into the middle of the slant-top. The grooves were smooth and cool, as Ma's hands had always felt, even at the end when she sat calmly in her favorite flowery chintz chair, eight flights above the bustle of East Seventy-fourth Street. Smaller, simpler scallops were carved into the middle of the three drawers below, each with brass handles that were mounted on brass plates reminiscent of tulips. The short feet were S-shaped. The desk was compact yet elegant, like Ma.

I began to relax about my own eventual end. I didn't want

it to come any time soon—please!—but Ma hadn't been afraid as she went through it. And whenever I wanted to be reassured by her graceful passing, I could sit here by her desk, hers and mine, that seemed to hold so much more closed than when I opened it.

I flipped the slant top down, located a notebook and pen, and wrote out exactly how I wanted my savings distributed, effortlessly, with a sense of caring and appropriateness that seemed to flow straight from Ma's heart.

That left the fate of my things. Over the next few days, I called several relatives about the desk. They were all sorry but didn't think they'd have room for it. When I hung up in the downstairs hall after talking with my cousin Kathy, I burst into tears.

Jan was in the living room, sweeping ashes from the fireplace into a dustpan. "What's the matter?" He rushed to me.

"No one wants Ma's desk when I die," I cried. I'd never considered asking him. Why would he be interested? He'd never met Ma.

He wrapped his arms around me. "Susan, if you die before I do, I'm leaving your study exactly the way it is."

Oh, my darling, I'm your darling too, aren't I?

Sitting at Ma's desk a few nights later, I smiled as I recalled that many of her other lovely things—her dining table and chairs, china, her fur coat—were with other family and friends, giving them comfort and pleasure. I swiveled my chair around and scanned the books stuffed onto the white floor-to-ceiling shelves Jan had built for me on the opposite wall. Books were the only things I'd ever accumulated. I walked over, pulled out Anne Morrow Lindbergh's *Gift from the Sea* and flipped open the cover. "Sue, Answers without questions—look again and sea. Love, Peter" my brother had written. Scanning the shelves, I spotted a number of books that relatives and friends had given me through the years. I cherished them all. "Let's, you and I, go grow cabbages! With trowel, will travel," Jean urged in *The Spirit of Findhorn*, about the spiritual community in Scotland that grew huge vegetables and communed with vegetable spirits.

It took hours but I signed my name inside all my books, writing it below if someone had already written hers or his— provenance even for paperbacks. I wasn't sure who might want any of the volumes, but my heart warmed at the possibilities. I especially hoped someone I loved—or someone I didn't know—would like my 1985 twenty-two-volume off-brand encyclopedia with its upside-down covers, my beloved ninth edition of *Webster's Collegiate Dictionary* with its frayed binding mended with duct tape and all the books given to me by my family and friends. After I had signed awhile, I felt refreshingly free of myself, as if I were happily diffusing.

Perhaps this lightening up helped to loosen a heretofore stuck stance of mine as well. One morning, another dripping one, windy too, I decided to trek, by car to the LIRR, by the LIRR to Manhattan, by the subway to the Bronx, and then by foot, to Woodlawn Cemetery. (I didn't consider simply driving to the cemetery because with my skills at reading maps and signs, this alternative would have ended up being even more circuitous.) I wondered if I might possibly agree, after all, to Jan's and my "cremains," as Clarissa called them, being buried at Woodlawn some day.

After consulting a map in the cemetery office, I cinched the belt of my trench coat, pointed my pink umbrella into the wet wind and galumphed in my rubber boots along the asphalt roads. The grassy hills, cleared of their autumn leaves, were dotted with towering oaks, elms and birches, whose mostly bare branches filigreed the sky. Innumerable modest gravestones seemed almost integral to the bucolic. Unfortunately,

there were also obelisks higher than trees and many mauso-
leums larger than New York apartments. My companions, a
score of Canada geese, not the least bothered by these excesses
of unbridled arrogance, simply waddled along, nibbling the
grass, attentive to what was important to them. I decided to
take my cue from the geese.

About ten minutes later, I came upon an obelisk thrusting
only about fifteen feet into the sky, inscribed with HAVEN.
On either side, sat practically identical granite stones, all two
feet high, curved on top and polished in front, in two virtually *symmetrical* rows. Still, the family plot looked almost artistic under the reaching branches of a grand elm, with a finely
branched dogwood and the green of rhododendrons and aza-
leas in the back. I stood in front of Ma's stone. REGINA HA-
VEN PUGH CUMMINGS was chiseled in block letters below GRACE HAVEN PUGH, whom I'd never heard of. The
stark, sharp declaration of my mother's death, not a bit softened by eleven years of exposure, stabbed my heart. "Hello,
Ma," I whispered. No response.

The rain had reduced to a drizzle. I walked back and forth
along the rows of stones. The names were surprisingly read-
able, considering that some dated back well over a century.
Ma was the most recent addition. The "presence" of so many
other relatives, a number of them sharing a stone, as Ma did
with GRACE, was somehow consoling, even though I hadn't
known any of them except Ma's mother, REGINA CAHILL
PUGH, dear Nana. Ma had adored her father, THOMAS
PUGH, but he died before I was born. I did recognize a few
other names that Ma had mentioned through the years. Stones
remembering three INFANTS made my eyes pool.

Suddenly I was gripped by the thought that I'd be deserting
Ma, Nana too, if I weren't buried near them. And walking by
name after chiseled name, I began to feel a compelling connec-

tion with all the other people buried there as well, with everyone as a whole, as if I were a tiny missing piece to a panoramic puzzle that had finally slipped into place. I was born of an elaborate heritage—of the Pughs, who crossed the ocean from Wales; of the Havens of England and the Cahills of Ireland; of the Cummings, who ventured down from the Scottish Highlands; of a staggering sequence of this person moving here and meeting that person from there, of arrangements and attractions, couplings and births. No doubt there were squabbles along the way, and even separations such as between Ma and Daddy, but there was also a breathtaking amount of loving. And I would not be expanding the panorama with any births myself.

I ran my hand along the tops of the front row of stones until I reached Ma's and knelt in the muddy grass and kissed her name. It would be a profound honor to some day have Jan's and my names carved into one of these old, gray stones, that held together, however loosely, so much life.

It might be quite an adventure.

I kissed Ma's name again and started back home, slower than the geese.

But by the time I passed through the cemetery gate, I was almost fast walking. I had so much to do. I had to tell Jan we were now totally compatible. Maybe our ashes could even mingle in the same vase. Oops. Urn. I was finally ready to call a lawyer. And I had to study *Blithe Spirit*. I'd heard that a theater on Long Island was about to hold auditions for the play—a chance to do Madame! Hey, Ma, you think you could sweet-talk the director?

Acknowledgments

Thank you, thank you and thank you again to
Elaine Edelman
Karen Braziller
Roberta J. Buland, Editor
my wild and wonderful writer friends, especially
Katherine Pritchard, Carolyn Lewis and *Faith Kindness*
the multi-talented *Maureen Moore* at Booksmyth Press
and
Jan
for their inspiration, encouragement and support,
and many kisses to *Jan* for accepting my peripatetic
writing ways and for asking often but not too often,
"Did you finish it yet?"

Notes

In Chapter 9, I am indebted to Louise L. Hay, *You Can Heal Your Life*
(Santa Monica: Hay House, 1984), pp. 157, 159, 5.

Page 105, lyrics from "Scalloped Potatoes,"
a round composed by Emily Fox

COLOPHON

The font for this edition uses, for text and headings, Adobe Garamond Premier Pro, a digital font based on an original design by Claude Garamond (1480-1561), a French publisher and type designer. His font offered such elegance and legibility that it spawned many versions then and into the present. Adobe's digital version was created in 1989 by Robert Slimbach.

Made in the USA
Charleston, SC
27 October 2012